The Quicksand
of Agoraphobia:

A memoir of panic disorder

by

Diane Mengali

1

Published by
Bright Penny Press

Copyright © 2017 Diane Mengali
The Quicksand of Agoraphobia: A memoir of panic disorder

ISBN: 978-0-9996471-0-3
Library of Congress Control Number: 2017960682
Printed in the United States of America

The names of individuals have been changed in the
narrative.

For Ellen, my mentors, and my mother

We read to know we are not alone.
—C.S. Lewis

PART ONE

1947-1966

"Sometimes, to move forward you have to look at the past."

(advice found in a fortune cookie)

Vigilance

The earliest memories I can conjure up consist of pervasive and ambiguous feelings of fear and dread. I feared that something somewhere was wrong or about to go wrong. This amorphous and lurking fear became reality when I started kindergarten in 1947 at age five. For the first few weeks of school, I cried inconsolably on the way to school. On arrival, my mother had to drag me out of the car and up two flights of stairs to the classroom. Terrified and afraid to leave my mother, I begged her to stay with me. She tried to console me by pointing out all the kids who were excited to be there, but the sight of joy and excitement around me only amplified my fear and sadness. When my mother handed me over to the nun standing at the classroom door, I felt like I was being abandoned forever. For the rest of the school day, I sat huddled and sobbing, waiting for class to end. The relief brought by the end of the school day was only temporary. When one day ended, I began obsessing on the next.

My mother, baffled by my distressing behavior, asked the nun for advice. The nun advised my mother to ignore my sobbing pleas for rescue and they would stop. She was right. I eventually ran out of steam and was forced to accept that rescue was not an option. Though I stopped crying, the oppressive and amorphous fear persisted along with the feeling of abandonment. Until I reached third grade, I cried and whimpered on the way to school for the first two weeks of every new school year.

By second grade, I was riding my bike two miles to school, crying all the way and praying that some calamitous event would occur, forcing me to return home. No matter how bad something else might be, it could never compare to the relentless, inexplicable terror I felt on my way to school.

My mother never drove us to school unless the weather was bad. When I entered third grade and my brother, Ned, started first grade, it became my job to get him to and from school. I was small, my bike was small and he was big. He sat on the back fender rack of my bike and dragged his feet on the ground. Now, in addition to being sad and fearful, I was angry because I had to be responsible for him. It was not uncommon for Ned to be kept after school for talking in class, which meant I had to hang around the school until he was released. He was so naive he thought the teacher kept him because she liked him.

In 1950 I was eight; my brother was six, and my sister, Patty, was a few months past three. To help my mother, I took on the responsibility of keeping track of both of them after school and on weekends. Every evening before dinner, I gathered up their scattered toys and scoured the neighborhood and a nearby park to find my siblings. My brother liked to grab a loaf of bread and a small wicker chair and survey the neighborhood. He was fascinated by lawn mowers, so when he came upon someone cutting the grass, he sat on his chair, ate bread and watched. On Saturdays, when there was a lot of yard action, he spent most of the day moving from yard to yard and block to block. It was my job to find him and bring him home.

My sister was like a feral cat, sneaky and difficult to catch. Her favorite place was the sandbox in the park where I frequently found her standing naked and peeing. Patty possessed Houdini's escape skills. No matter how my mother tried to confine her, she always ended up free and loose in the neighborhood. Neighbors from blocks away called our house regularly to inform us of her location. It was then my job to fetch her. Baffled by my sister's ability to escape, my mother and I searched the yard for clues. Under the neighbor's flimsy fence, we found a carved out, toddler size opening which allowed my sister to slither under the fence into the neighbor's back yard. From there, she escaped into the neighborhood by way of their gate. My mother plugged every possible exit hole but nothing worked. My sister was cunning and determined.

I became obsessively vigilant and responsible. My brother did risky things like pile up chairs in the kitchen and climb on them to reach my mother's stash of money. There was a grocery bus that came through the neighborhood weekly, and my brother would climb up on the counter to reach money for a treat. His treat-buying ended when he fell and broke a collarbone. I found him lying in pain on the kitchen floor.

My mother was never in the room when a catastrophe hit. She read constantly and spent hours with the neighbor on the other side of our duplex reading and discussing books. She read to satisfy her brilliant and curious mind and to escape from reality and the mindless drudgery of housework. Believing that children, like zucchini, grew and flourished with sunshine and very little oversight, she permitted us to behave like uncaged animals until my father came home from work. Before his arrival, my mother scurried around with a dust cloth and the vacuum cleaner trying to make the house look like she'd been cleaning all day. She depended on me to help her restore order.

My father owned a men's clothing store that had been started by his father, an Italian immigrant who was a shoemaker. My father disliked retail but felt a filial obligation to keep the business going. When business was slow or the customers annoying, he'd come home in a bad mood. I always tried to read my father's mood so I could brace myself for the fallout. Sometimes he'd yell at us kids, but my mother was usually his victim. If my father came home to a dirty house or unruly children, he criticized my mother mercilessly, guaranteeing an unpleasant dinner experience. After one of my father's attacks, I saw my mother's hands shake so badly she could hardly pick up a fork. When dinner was over, I did my homework at the cleared dinner table. From where I sat I could see my mother washing dishes. On the nights when my father had verbally attacked her, I watched helplessly as the tears fell from her eyes into the dishwater. I wanted to help her but didn't know what to do. I wanted her to get mad, but she remained passively silent. On those evenings, I went to bed sad for my mom and angry at my father. I was eight years old but I was quickly learning to read my father's mood and my mother's level of anxiety.

During the summer of 1950, my job as mother's helper became more demanding. My parents, who sometimes partied with friends on Saturday nights, slept late on Sundays. Since my sister and I shared a room, I knew when she crawled out of bed early on Sunday mornings that she was looking for food and people. When she found neither, she foraged for herself. One Sunday, after hearing her open and shut several cupboards in the kitchen, I got up to find her sitting on the living room floor in a mound of Tide. She looked quite content shoving fistfuls of the detergent into her mouth. I banged frantically on my parents' bedroom door yelling for help. My father, annoyed and disheveled, opened the door to the Tide scene. "My God. What in the hell is Patty eating?"

I said, "She's eating Tide, Dad. She got it out of the kitchen. There's a trail of it leading from the kitchen to the living room."

"Go in and wake your mother. Tell her what's happened while I clean up this kid."

"Mom, wake up! It's important! Patty ate Tide and dad needs you."

My mother threw on her robe and ran into the living room.

"Oh my God! That stuff is toxic. We need to get her to a hospital. She needs her stomach pumped."

Both parents dressed hurriedly and ran out of the house carrying Patty. I stayed home with my sleeping brother and cleaned up the mess.

On another Sunday not long afterward, with the aid of a chair, my sister managed to climb within reach of the medicine cabinet in the bathroom. I found her sitting on the floor polishing off a bottle of baby aspirin. By the time my sister was four, her stomach had been pumped out twice.

One weekday during that same summer, my mother was outside sunbathing and reading a book. I had been instructed to watch my siblings, who were playing in my parents' bedroom. Since they were quietly coloring, I went into another room to read a book. When the quiet had gone on too long, I checked on them only to discover that they had drawn all over the white bedroom walls with one of my mother's lipsticks. While I was surveying the damage, my brother let out a piercing scream. He was sitting on the floor with a bobby pin shoved into one opening of an electrical plug. He couldn't let go because he was frozen to the outlet. The scream brought my mother into the room. When she saw my brother, she ordered us not to touch him. She grabbed a heavy blanket, threw it around him, and pulled him away from the plug. With the exception of a blistered arm, he was unscathed.

On seeing the crimson-smeared walls, my mother came apart. She feared that my father would come home before she had time to clean up the mess. With great urgency, she and I scrubbed the walls, removing most of the mess. She asked me over and over, "Do you think he'll notice? What am I going to do? How do I explain your brother's arm? I'll have to make up something that won't make him mad or I'll never hear the end of it. What do you think I should say?"

Other than helping her by rounding up toys and siblings, I had no idea how to help her with my father. After the coloring incident, I began to see my mother differently. In my child's mind and heart, I sensed a sadness and fragility in her that frightened me. My vigilance increased as I understood more clearly how much my mother depended on me. Being responsible for my siblings and helping my mother restore order were ways of protecting her. I wasn't just helping her, I was saving her. At the same time I was clinging to her on the school steps, she was looking for her own life raft. We both needed the same things: kindness, understanding, and protection. As a kid, I did what I could for my mother because I was afraid not to. I clung to her and tried to protect her in order to save both of us. What I couldn't foresee at age eight was that my obsessive need to protect my mother would set me up for a lifetime of putting her needs before mine.

Housewarming

In the summer of 1951, my family moved across town into a brand-new house. It was a large ranch-style home with a big backyard. My father was ecstatic. Filled with enthusiasm, he could hardly wait to plant the yard and settle in. My mother seemed tentative and withdrawn, as if she were afraid of the house. On occasion she'd say, "I really miss the old duplex. It was small and cozy. I especially miss Dorothy, our old neighbor. She was so smart and funny. Now I won't have anyone to read or laugh with."

My father, irritated by her lack of enthusiasm would say, "I don't understand why you seem so unhappy. Many women would give anything to move into a house like this."

After we settled into our home, my mother became severely depressed. She began moping around the house, convinced she was dying. She spent her days lying on the couch, barely able to get dinner on the table. When I asked her what was wrong, her answer was always, "I don't know, but I think I'm dying. I think I have cancer or a heart problem but I won't go to any of the local quacks. They don't know anything. I need to go to UC San Francisco or Stanford Medical School."

When she talked about dying, I believed her. But when I asked my father about her, he'd say, "There's nothing wrong with your mother. She's just a hypochondriac, someone pretending to be sick so she doesn't have to do housework or help me plant the new yard. Your mother comes from a crazy, intellectual family who believes housework is beneath them. Look at your grandmother. She's a career woman who lives in an apartment in San Francisco. When we visit, there's never any food in the place and she never does housework." My father would rant on about my mother's family and how screwed up they were until she screamed at him or started crying. Then he would attack her for being a lousy cook and housekeeper. She usually ended up going to her bedroom and staying there until my father ordered her to get dinner on the table.

I worried about my mother almost constantly. Her behavior, never very explicable, became even stranger. One afternoon when it was over 100 degrees, my mother sat in the back yard watching my father plant shrubs. She was wearing her heaviest winter coat and looked like she was about to cry. I thought that anyone who needed to wear such a heavy coat during the summer must surely be sick. Every night when I went to bed I wondered how long my mother would live and what I would do without her.

As the summer went on, so did my mother's depression. My father finally agreed to take her to Stanford for a medical workup. She stayed there for a week and was declared to be in perfect health. My mother doubted their assessment and went to UC San Francisco for another opinion. Their assessment was the same as Stanford's with one difference: she needed to see a psychiatrist, which my father took as proof she was crazy. She was referred to a doctor in San Francisco. Dad made fun of her for needing to see a "shrink," and complained bitterly about how much "this craziness" was going to cost him.

When school started in the fall of 1951, I was delighted. I was in the fifth grade and would turn ten in October. With the move, the Catholic school I'd been attending was just a few blocks away, and I no longer had to supervise my siblings. We rode our bikes separately and seldom saw each other at school. The playground was divided by age groups and God help you if you stepped over any lines. The nuns were strict, but the structure that the rules provided made me feel safe. After school and on weekends, I'd usually ride my bike to a friend's house. This escape, along with reading, provided distraction from the problems at home.

That fall, my mother took the bus to San Francisco for her weekly appointment with the psychiatrist. Since the return bus didn't arrive until after dinner, we went to my paternal grandmother's after school. We either ate there, or my father would take us to a diner across from the bus station. I was always glad to see my mother come off the bus. But on the way home, my father tormented her. "Did you tell the shrink the truth? Did you tell him that you hated housework and that I washed windows? No man should have to work all week and then spend his weekends washing windows. Did you tell him about your crazy family?" My mother cried. We kids cried, and I screamed at my father to stop picking on mom. He would pull over to the curb so he could reach into the back seat and slap whatever part of me he could reach. Then he started in on my mother again. "See, this is all your fault. If you were normal like other women, I wouldn't be wasting my money on a shrink. Are you satisfied now that everyone is upset?" The two miles from the bus station to home seemed like twenty. When we got there, my mother sat sobbing in the living room while I tried to console her.

After five visits, my mother quit going. On our last ride home from the bus station, my mother told my father, "Do you know what Dr. Wilson said today? He told me that the wrong person in the family was seeing him."

My father sneered. "After that remark, I shouldn't pay that bastard. Besides, you haven't changed. He hasn't done a thing for you. This has all been a waste of time and money."

But after her last session, my mother became more engaged and assertive. I didn't know what was going on inside her, but she seemed more "normal." She cooked and did housework just like my friends' mothers. If my father complained about her cooking, she threatened to throw his dinner away. My father started to complain less. Things were going smoother, and I felt I could stop worrying about her.

16

The Christmas of 1951 was our first Christmas in the new house. That holiday was a Norman Rockwell portrait of normalcy. During the break from school, I spent most days at my father's store. He gave me a job folding boxes for five cents apiece. The boxes varied in size: one for neckties, shirts, and sweaters. I was a compulsively fast box-folder with fingers sporting Band-Aids to cover paper cuts. When there was a backlog of completed boxes, I'd sit on the floor in front of a space-heater and read a *Bobbsey Twins* book. Sometimes, I'd sit at my father's desk to draw or to pretend I was a business owner. In the late afternoon, with a pocketful of nickels, I'd go next door to Woolworth's to Christmas shop.

It was thrilling to be downtown during Christmas. The four retail blocks of Main Street were decorated and Christmas music floated out of every store. The business owners formed a tightly-knit community, and when there was a lull in business, the owners would wander into each other's stores to chat and to compare sales. On a box-folding break, I'd roam around downtown to check out the other stores' decorations and merchandise.

On Christmas eve, my dad closed early so our family could have an early dinner at the Hotel Woodland, located a block away from his store. It was an old hotel with a large lobby, a nice garden, a bar, a formal dining room and a coffee shop. It was rumored that Clark Gable had stayed there while in the area on a hunting trip. We always ate in the coffee shop where we'd eat fast and race home to open presents. My father, excited over our new house, insisted that Christmas Eve be moved from my grandparents' house to ours. Before we could dig into the presents, we had to wait until my aunt, uncle and cousins arrived from San Francisco. After everyone's arrival, we were handed our presents by a family friend dressed as Santa. On Christmas day, family and friends went to my grandmother's for an incredible Italian feast.

In the spring of 1952, my mother decided she was bored at home and wanted to work at my father's menswear' store. My father asked her who was going to clean house and be home for the kids after school. Her solution was to hire someone to do these things. In a discussion between my parents about the store, I heard my mother admit that she was becoming afraid to stay home alone and needed to be with my father. When my father asked my mom why she couldn't be alone, she said, "I don't know. I just get nervous being home alone." Sometimes when she talked about it, her hands shook.

My mom pleaded with my father to let her work at the store. Her plan was to replace an employee and pay for the hired housekeeper with the savings. After many heated arguments and soulful pleadings, my father gave in. My parents hired Carmen, a Mexican lady with twelve kids of her own. She stayed with us after school and throughout the summer of 1952. I loved her. She was warm, jovial and calm—a welcome respite from my parents.

The Glass Scare

By the time I entered the sixth grade, I was well on my way to becoming a chronic worrier. When school started, my mother quit working at my dad's store. Now that she was home during the day, I worried about how she was managing home alone. While I was supposed to be paying attention in class, I found my mind drifting, trying to picture the scene at home. Was my mother reading, vacuuming, moping or crying? The teacher always brought me back to reality by calling on me to answer a question that rendered me speechless. I daydreamed often and found myself conjuring up frightening scenarios that might be happening at home. I was relieved when I came home to find my mother cooking, cleaning or reading.

A few months into the school year, I had a scare that intensified my chronic state of worry. One day during lunch, my teacher called me aside to ask if I had drunk the milk from my thermos. When I told her that I had, she became flustered. Turns out my mother had called the school in a panic to tell them not to let me drink my milk, because the milk bottle she'd used to fill my thermos was chipped. When I got home, my mother expressed concern that I might have swallowed slivers of glass. She had called the doctor who told her to watch for internal bleeding. For days I watched and waited for blood to come gushing out of either end of my body. As a result of this scare, I refused to eat or drink from anything made of glass. To accommodate my need to avoid glass, my mother bought me a plastic dish and glass which sat at my place at the table.

I became so obsessed with the fear of swallowing broken glass that for two years I ate only from paper or plastic plates. I refused to eat or drink anything away from home that didn't meet this criterion. My father, who thought the situation absurd, blamed my mother for scaring me and then giving in to my fear and avoidance by buying plastic plates and glasses. His solution was to let me go hungry until my only option was to eat off regular plates. His other "cure" for the problem was to embarrass me. Any time a friend or relative showed up at meal time, he'd point out that I ate out of a plastic "dog bowl."

Due mostly to embarrassment and inconvenience, I gradually weaned myself off the plastic by thinking differently. I told myself that before the thermos scare, I had eaten off glass for years and nothing bad had happened. I also thought that if it were easy to die from glass plates and glasses, no one would be eating off them. I worked hard on my thinking for two years before I could throw away the plastic. But for many years after "fixing" myself, I still avoided plates with chips and cracks and I always ran my finger around the rim of a glass looking for chips. Eventually, even the chips and cracks became irrelevant.

Though the glass issue produced stress and fear, the cause of the fear could be attributed to a specific object, making it easier to overcome. During the time I avoided glass, I realized that my response to the situation was extreme and irrational, but knowing this didn't stop me from reacting irrationally. My extreme reaction was beyond my control. It was like a switch in my head had tripped as a response to overload. Though I was able to overcome the glass scare, my reaction to the scare was a harbinger of the avoidance behavior that would occur much later.

Lake Tahoe

For two weeks every summer, my dad rented a house at Lake Tahoe. He'd taken the family to the west shore of Tahoe every summer since we were small. We all loved the lake, especially my father, who dreamed of owning a place there. For those two weeks, everyone was relaxed and happy. During the day, Ned, Patty and I played in the ice-cold lake. On emerging, we covered ourselves with Coppertone, spread our towels on the warm pier and sunbathed. While lying on the pier, I'd close my eyes to absorb the smells I associated with the lake: the pine, the Coppertone and the varnished wood of the pier. Even the fuel smell emanating from the gorgeous wooden boats tied to the pier seemed memorable. Then, I focused on the sounds: the small waves lapping at the pier, the start of a wooden boat's powerful engine, the sound of crunching rocks as people walked by on the beach, and the chipmunks scampering up and down the pines.

We seldom went to Tahoe without guests. My parents' friends, many of whom had kids, took turns driving up to stay for a few days. Sometimes, my grandparents came along as vacationers and babysitters. One couple with three kids whose ages matched ours, stayed with us for a week most summers. They owned a beautiful boat and every day, all of us kids hounded the poor man for boat rides and water-ski tows. In the evenings, if the adults went to the casinos, all the kids would be dropped off at a movie theater showing a double-feature. The parents would always be waiting for us after the movie.

In the summer of 1953, two of my parents' best friends came with us to Tahoe. Both were eccentric, smart, and witty bachelors who liked to party. Their names were Al and Marty. Al was a third grade teacher in Sacramento and Marty was the head librarian at the California State Law Library in Sacramento. Before her marriage to my father, my mother had met Al through a friend of hers in Sacramento, while my father had met Marty during his years studying at UC Berkeley. Marty had finished his B.A. in library science at Stanford, and was getting his master's at Cal. My father had been in his senior year at Cal, finishing his B.A. in history. Both men were like family; they were always around. When they rode to Tahoe with us, Al brought sandwiches, cookies and sodas. We ate in the car on the way, which annoyed my father who yelled at us about getting food crumbs all over the car. Al, who was easy-going and liked kids, was one of the few people who consistently laughed at my father while telling him to "shut up."

During Marty and Al's stay, there was no baby-sitter available, which left my parents pondering how the four of them could escape to the casinos. My father came up with a simple plan for the first escape. "We can drop the kids off at the miniature golf course in Kings Beach. It's on the way to the casinos and it stays open late. We'll eat dinner early so we'll have plenty of time to gamble." Then he asked us kids, "Would you like to play miniature golf at Kings Beach while we're at the casinos?"

The three of us answered excitedly. "Yeah, we like to go there."

"Well, now's your chance. You can spend the whole evening there."

We arrived at the golf course at 6:00. My father gave us enough money to buy snacks and play all evening. He checked the closing time of 10:00 and promised to be back by then. After two hours of golf, we were tired and bored, but still had two hours to go before pickup. At 10:00 sharp, the manager turned off all the lights and told us to wait in front of the entrance. Figuring my parents were on the way, I tried to stay calm by telling myself they'd arrive any minute. At 11:00, we were still standing by the highway, looking hopefully at every car that came around the curve in the road. Now, it was getting cold and we were sleepy. I was terrified, but tried to look calm while I obsessed on disastrous possibilities. *I wonder if they forgot about us? They've never been late before. Maybe they're in an accident. How are we going to get home? What if they never show up?*

I noticed a well-lit motel next to the golf course. There was a large wooden swing out in front where we went to sit down. The clock in the motel's office read 11:15. At 11:30, the innkeeper came out and said, "Are you kids all right?

What are you doing up this late? How old are you anyway? Are you staying at the motel?"

I spoke. "No. We're not staying here and we're eleven, nine and seven. My parents dropped us off at the golf course next door and promised to pick us up by closing. We're still waiting for them."

"Do you know where they are? I could call them for you."

"They're at the casinos."

"Well, I'd have to call all the casinos and have them paged. They'll probably be here soon. You could wait inside the office where it's warmer. I hope they get here before midnight. I turn the outside lights off then."

Now I really panicked. "I think we better wait outside where my parents can see us. Otherwise, they won't know where we are."

A few minutes before midnight, my parents rolled up. We ran for the car. When I got in, I said, "Where were you? We've been waiting since ten when the golf course closed. I was afraid something bad had happened."

My father said, "I thought the golf course closed at eleven. I must've read the sign wrong. We were all gambling and winning and just lost track of time. This won't happen again."

Then Al chimed in, "Your dad was really on a roll at the craps table. He walked away two-hundred dollars ahead. The rest of us were winning on the slots and didn't want to leave. I'll make you some hot chocolate when we get home."

The next morning, the adults were tired and hung-over. I ate some cereal and went out to the pier to read. Angry and scared, I was thinking about being "dumped" last night and whether I could trust my parents again.

For the next several evenings after the golf incident, the adults took turns staying home with us. Sometimes, my parents took us to a nice restaurant for dinner. At least one night during our yearly stay, they took us to a dinner show at a casino where headliners such as Liberace and Tony Bennett performed.

On the evenings when we actually stayed home with our parents, we walked together on the beach, then sat at the end of the pier to watch the sun set over the lake. After dark, we played cards and board games. During these evenings, I felt happy and safe.

A few days before the end of our vacation, my parents, Marty and Al wanted to visit the casinos together again, which meant finding a place to leave us. My parents picked Tahoe Tavern resort. We loved "The Tavern" as it was called by the locals. Built in 1901, it was a magnificent, opulent 225-room, four-story hotel located just outside Tahoe City. It had a waterfront boardwalk, one of Tahoe's longest piers, plush lawns and rock-lined walkways that traversed the extensive grounds. Inside the main building was a massive, well-appointed lobby and a luxurious dining room, reserved for the hotel guests. A separate building housed a soda fountain, barbershop, a movie theater and a bowling alley. A large swimming pool and tennis courts offered additional recreational opportunities. A full-service laundry, a doctor's office and a steam plant sat on the far side of the grounds. The long, winding, tree-lined entrance to the hotel ended next to a set of long-abandoned railroad tracks. In the early days, hotel guests could take a train from Truckee to the Tavern.

The splendor of the Tavern fascinated me. The public could pay to use the swimming pool, the bowling alley or see a movie. My parents took us there often to swim and bowl. A swim, a sandwich at the soda fountain, and a walk on the pier made for a perfect day. Sometimes, instead of swimming, we'd bowl all afternoon. When we had guests with kids staying with us and all the adults went gambling, the movie theater at the Tavern served as our baby-sitter.

While the structure and setting of the Tavern was like something out of a dream, something that was too large or mythical to absorb or grab hold of, the guests presented their own intrigue. Compared to the wealthy, well-dressed hotel patrons, the day guests looked like street urchins from a Dickens' novel. There was an implied line of demarcation that physically separated the wealthy guests from the day-trippers. The expansive front lawn, the covered porch lined with tables and chairs, the lobby and dining room belonged exclusively to the hotel guests. While lounging around the pool, I loved to watch the guests. The women wore hats and expensive dresses and sipped colorful drinks. The men, who gathered separately from the women, wore white slacks or summer suits and smoked cigars. Even their children were dressed up during the day, with the girls in dresses and the boys wearing suits and ties. I'd only seen people like this in movies and I wondered how any of them could have fun while dressed in such restrictive clothing.

Because I'd spent so many enjoyable days at the Tavern, I felt comfortable when my parents announced they were leaving us there while they gambled. My father gave us enough money to eat at the soda fountain, go to the movies and bowl. The show was the last venue to close, and my father promised to be there when the show got out at 11:00.

Our first stop was the soda fountain, where we gulped down sandwiches, and sodas and filled our pockets with candy. Anxious to get a lane before the bowling alley got crowded, we headed there next. An hour into bowling, my sister, Patty, got into a fight over the only small bowling ball in the place. She and one of the suit and tie kids from the hotel tried to beat each other to the ball as it came up the ball return. My sister usually won. As soon as the boy's mother appeared, he started crying and pointing to my sister. The mother complained to the manager, who ordered us to leave.

We went upstairs to the theater and bought our tickets. We were early, therefore had our choice of seats. The theater was directly above the bowling alley and we could hear the pins being knocked down and reset. We could also hear the pin boys talking and laughing. Once the movie started, the annoying bowling sounds were replaced by clouds of cigar and cigarette smoke swirling in front of the screen. About half-way through the second feature, a swarm of bats flew in somewhere in the roof above the projection room. They darted around just below the ceiling of the huge theater. Startled and frightened, all the patrons fled and the projector shut down.

With all the other venues closed, there was nothing to do but wait for our parents. Thankfully, it was almost their promised arrival time of 11:00. We stood under a green, metal outdoor light that was attached to the building housing the bowling alley. The building faced the entrance road and we could see the headlights of cars rounding the curve to the hotel. While we were waiting, a creepy-looking janitor started sweeping the sidewalks around the buildings. When he saw us, he stopped, leaned on his broom and stared. We waited for him to say something, but he just kept staring. Finally, he started sweeping again, but he swept slowly and mechanically, with his gaze fixed on us.

I was terrified, but tried to look nonchalant. I could see the hotel from where we stood, and thought about running into the lobby. This possibility for escape quickly dwindled as I watched the lobby lights and several exterior lights go out. It was now midnight and we were huddled beneath the light with the creepy-sweeper for company.

Though it was late, cars were still coming up the long driveway to the hotel. Every time we saw a set of headlights bounce off the trees, we said hopefully, "Here they come. This has to be them." I was on the verge of tears when my parents showed up at 12:30. The conversation that ensued was a repeat of the miniature golf episode; the parents were winning money and had lost track of time.

I was hurt, angry and scared. *How could my parents have so little concern for our feelings? Why didn't they keep their promises?* I was too afraid of my dad to ask him these questions.

That summer, I was glad to get back home where I had more control over my life. I could come and go on my bike as I pleased. I was still angry about being "dumped" twice while my parents gambled. The fear that I felt on those nights had rekindled the feelings of panic and abandonment that had plagued me as a younger school girl.

Helplessness and Despair

I never knew exactly when my mother crossed the line between social drinking and alcoholism, but in the summer of 1954, I noticed a significant change in her relationship with alcohol. Until that summer, I had been unaffected by the amount of alcohol people consumed. Because I had grown up around drinkers, I considered drinking to be a normal activity. My parents liked to party on weekends and would sometimes have a beer or highball before dinner on weeknights. Many of my friends' parents had drinks every night before dinner. My Italian grandfather drank a bottle or more of wine a day. Every summer my parents hosted large outdoor parties and when I saw people drunk at these parties, I considered their intoxication a temporary state, not a sign of a larger problem.

When my parents gave parties, my dad set up the yard and my mother cooked. On many of these occasions, my mother started her cooking tasks in a sober state, but by the time dinner was ready to be carried outside, she had developed a stagger that made carrying large trays of food a perilous task. Some of the female guests and I would rush to her aid and relieve her of the food trays. The nights when she started out this way, by the end of the party she was so drunk that she fell into bed, leaving the dirty dishes for the next day. My father, who couldn't stand messes, always cleaned up the yard after the party and expected my mother to wash the massive pile of dishes and clean up the kitchen. When he found her passed out in the bedroom, he'd be furious. Whether he did the dishes or left them for my mother, he berated her for days about the mess she left.

After a few of these ugly party scenes, I wondered how my mother was getting so drunk. Since she didn't drink very much during the party, I wondered when she was drinking. At the next opportunity, I made it a point to observe her surreptitiously. I discovered that while she was cooking, she'd pause occasionally and reach for a bottle of liquor that was hidden behind a large can of olive oil under the sink. I watched her as she took big swigs from the bottle during the entire time she cooked. My heart sank when I saw this. I didn't know what to do. I couldn't tell my father because I knew he would berate her. I decided that the only thing I could do was watch her every time my parents entertained. If I could judge her level of intoxication by her behavior, maybe I could discover a way to prevent disaster. The task of keeping my mother sober would require that I maintain a high degree of vigilance as well as the ability to distract her. Since she wouldn't drink in front of me, when she cooked for guests I stayed in the kitchen talking to her and helping her. Because I was the only one aware of her clandestine drinking, I felt the need to save her from herself and from my father's wrath.

In the fall of 1955, when I started eighth grade, my mother was once again struggling with bouts of deep depression. Trying to assess her state of mind was one of the first things I did when I arrived home from school. If mom was depressed, I would warn my siblings that she was "in a funk." This was code for "we're in for a bad evening." When my mother was depressed, my father got angry and picked on her at dinner. He complained about her cooking and enumerated her faults. His cruel and critical behavior continued throughout dinner. By the time he finished his dinner, my mother would be shaking and sobbing. Without a thought for my mother's feelings, my father would bolt from the table while I stayed to console her. Between sobs she'd say, "That man treats me terribly. I can't do anything right. All he does is criticize me. I don't deserve this. Some days I wish I were dead." When she calmed down, I helped her with the dishes, then tried to concentrate on my homework.

Several weeks into the school year, my mother developed a strange, new behavior characterized by slurred words, rapidly blinking eyes and a visible struggle to appear normal. Normally, when I came home from school, she was either depressed and lying on the couch or she was doing housework and cooking dinner. Now when I came home from school, I didn't know which mother I would find. I hoped for the funny, good-humored, intelligent mother who would be fixing dinner. Sometimes I found the depressed mother. But other times, I found this new mother, the slurred mother I didn't understand. Then over time I made some discoveries: For one, I saw her drinking again from the bottle hidden behind the olive oil. Then I happened on an empty bottle while playing on the couch. I wondered why it was there but passed it off as some freak thing and threw it away.

One morning while racing around trying to get ready for school on time, I discovered that I didn't have a clean, ironed school blouse in my closet. We wore uniforms at the Catholic school and were expected to show up in clean, freshly ironed clothes. I panicked when I saw no blouse and ran to look for one in the ironing basket on the back porch. While rummaging through the basket and praying for a clean blouse, I found an empty liquor bottle hidden in the clothes. As I ironed my blouse, I cried. When I finished ironing, I buried the bottle in the basket and rushed to school, crying all the way. I arrived late. When the teacher scolded me in front of the class, I sobbed. My tardiness and tears earned me two hours of detention.

I didn't know what to do or whom to tell about my mother's drinking. Once again, I began my watch. Even though she didn't drink every night, I still watched, believing that by staying alert I could avert any potential disaster. On the days when she did drink, I prayed that her slight stagger and slurred words would go unnoticed by my self-absorbed father.

Soon after I discovered the empty bottles, my mother's drinking spiraled out of control. By the time I got home from school, she'd already be drunk. My brother and I could measure her degree of intoxication by how rapidly she blinked her eyes. Whoever got home first from school would assess the situation then communicate my mother's status through slow or fast eye blinks. My siblings and I spent many afternoons watching television and watching my mother guzzle whiskey while she cooked.

By dinner, she'd usually be too drunk to eat. If she managed to sit upright through the meal, my father would attack her relentlessly. "You're a disgusting drunk. You're ruining this family. You've never been a good wife or mother. You make me sick. Get out of my sight." My mother would either stagger off to her bedroom or sit at the table and sob, slurring out the words, "I wish I were dead. It would be better for everyone if I were dead." When I tried to defend or protect her by telling my father to leave her alone, he'd threaten to hit me. Once when I told him I hated him, he whipped me so hard with a belt I could barely sit still in school.

The angrier my father became and the more he nagged my mother, the more she drank and the less work she did. He tried to control her drinking by hiding the liquor but my mother always managed to get alcohol, usually by skimping on groceries and saving the excess money for booze.

Though my mother had serious problems, I knew she was basically a good person who needed help and support. Never once did my father utter a kind word to her. Never once did I see him console, hug or make any attempt to offer her support or help. He responded to her neediness and pleas for help by blaming her and beating her down. His behavior enraged me and made me ever more determined to protect my mother, a role I had been groomed for since early childhood. As I struggled to help her, I began to feel a heavy sadness that weighed me down.

I dragged this sadness around like a ball and chain. Even when I was having fun with friends, the sadness never left; it just retreated to the back of my mind.

In addition to the sadness, I was developing some peculiar, uncontrollable behaviors which added to my anxiety. I turned light switches off and on a set number of times on entering and leaving a room. I avoided cracks in the sidewalk. I hung and re-hung my clothes. My bed had to be made a certain way. Though I found the need for counting and repeating prescribed activities annoying, stressful and time-consuming, I couldn't stop it. The repetitive behavior seemed to be attached to some kind of magic and served as a talisman. My mind told me that if I turned the light switch off and on twenty times, nothing bad would happen that day. But if I ignored the impulse, bad things were guaranteed to happen. I had no idea what was happening to me or how to stop it but I thought my brain was shorting out. With no other options, I just lived with it and eventually it became like a constant, low-level background noise.

I was also lonely. In the 1950s, nobody discussed family problems. My embarrassed father insisted that my mother's drinking remain a secret. I was miserable. Completely, unrelentingly miserable. Then I met Miss Simpson.

Miss Simpson

A few weeks into eighth grade, I was asked to go steady by a boy I had a crush on. When I accepted, Mike presented me with a large, heavy-chained, ID bracelet engraved with his name. I wore this proof of adolescent devotion on my skinny wrist. Our dating life consisted of holding hands in Saturday matinees and close-dancing at occasional dance parties. This seemingly solid, simplistic and normal pattern of early teenage romance provided comfort, acceptance and a sense of sexual identity. That heavy ID bracelet was a social and sexual anchor, keeping me moored in a safe, familiar place.

As eighth graders in 1956, we had access to several movie magazines such as *Photoplay* and *Silver Screen*. These magazines contained full page, frame-ready pictures of the stars. The girls drooled over the likes of Tony Curtis, Troy Donahue and Tab Hunter. I wasn't boy-crazy like some of the girls, but I did like boys. While I thought these guys were darling, I found myself staring at Sophia Loren and falling madly in love with Audrey Hepburn.

One morning while playing dodge ball before class, I saw a new teacher who resembled Audrey Hepburn in looks and demeanor. I froze in place staring at her. My heart went places it had never gone before. Here in my midst was someone as beautiful as Audrey. She had perfect skin, high cheekbones, large brown eyes, a perfect nose and full lips. Her broad smile radiated warmth. I couldn't stop thinking about this teacher, and I knew on some instinctual level that I couldn't share my excitement with anyone. Girls were only supposed to be this excited about boys. Despite these confusing concerns, I was determined to find a way to get close to Audrey's twin, Miss Anne Simpson, the new first grade teacher.

Several weeks into the school year, the principal announced that the eighth graders who scored high in math or spelling could skip those classes two days a week in exchange for helping out in the lower grades. I qualified to skip spelling if I helped the first graders with reading and spelling. So I volunteered and soon found myself in Miss Simpson's classroom sitting like a giant in a first-grade desk. My job was to help with phonics, but I was constantly distracted by Miss Simpson's presence. Just being in the same room with her made my heart pound; I fought the urge to stare at her. When she sat next to me or inadvertently touched me, every inch of my body tingled. A soothing warmth and kindness radiated from her, and whatever balm she seemed to possess, I needed its healing power.

Desperate for more time with her, I offered to help her with chores after school and on weekends. We spent many afternoons and Saturdays covering books and fixing up her classroom. And we talked. Our conversations had been casual until the day she said, "You seem so sad. Is something wrong? You can tell me about it. Maybe I can help."

When she tapped into my sadness, it was like a dam inside me broke. I cried, and cried as she sat there patiently. Finally, I spoke. "My mother is drunk most days when I get home from school and my father is mean to her. I feel sorry for my mother and wish I could help her."

She listened intently then said, "Your mother needs kindness and support right now. You can't stop her from drinking but maybe you could help her by doing things around the house. On nights she can't do the dishes, you could do them for her. This would make both of you feel better. Please don't hate your mother because she drinks. Your mother needs help. You must be strong and have faith that your mother will get better." Riding home on my bike, I'd replay our conversations in my head. When the house was quiet at night, I tried to recapture the soothing warmth I felt when I was with Miss Simpson.

I learned that I could trust her with my feelings. I could cry or be frightened and she'd comfort me. Her kindness and understanding replaced my father's judgment and scolding. In contrast to the chaos in my home, I found acceptance and peace in her presence. No matter how bad things got at home, I knew I could survive because I had a safe place where my spirit could thrive. Miss Simpson became my mentor and my anchor. At the end of the school year when my classmates were thrilled about graduating and going to high school, I was devastated. Miss Simpson was leaving town for the summer and I was bereft, crying clandestinely for weeks. Somehow I survived the summer.

I had agreed to help Miss Simpson ready her classroom when she returned in August. When she arrived, I raced out to her classroom where we spent several glorious days unpacking boxes. We talked with an ease that a summer apart did nothing to interrupt. She still radiated peace, warmth and gentleness. Whenever we sat in silence, I could feel her peacefulness flow out and cover me like a soft, protective blanket. Sometimes while we were quiet, she'd smile at me and I would feel that important but indefinable messages passed between us in that silence.

Though Miss Simpson seemed like an ethereal being, I knew she was a mortal with a history. I wanted to know more about her life, so I started with a simple question. "I was wondering if you grew up in California?"

"Yes, as a matter of fact, I was born and raised in southern California."

Sensing my curiosity about her life, she continued. "I was born there twenty-three years ago, which makes me ten years older than you."

"This is your first year in Woodland. Are you going to stay here for a while?"

"I may stay here a few more years. My goal is to become a Catholic missionary somewhere in Asia. During the summer, I take language classes and learn about different countries."

Things were going so well, I asked about her parents. "Do your parents still live in southern California?"

There was a long, sad silence before she answered. "My father still lives there. My mother died a tragic death when I was about your age. Her death, especially the way she died, really devastated my family."

Her words hung in the air. I remained silent. There were no more questions to be asked.

I was stunned, but made a feeble attempt to express a sympathy that reflected my limited, adolescent understanding of death.

I dwelled on Miss Simpson's revelation about her mother and wondered if something so dreadful could have helped Miss Simpson become a kind, beautiful person. She had told me many times, "If we make the best of things we can't change, we become stronger people." Then, I wondered if her experience with her mother had made her more empathetic to my situation. Perhaps she saw me as the frightened child she had been at my age.

With the start of high school, the time I spent with Miss Simpson was limited to light homework days and free weekends. That June, we parted again and I cried. To escape the void created by Miss Simpson's absence, I immersed myself in a summer spent swimming with friends and dating my boyfriend, Mike.

Throughout high school, I continued to visit Miss Simpson often. Life at home had not improved and I still needed the safety and comfort of her presence. The year

I finished high school, Miss Simpson left town to fulfill her dream of becoming a missionary. I knew I would miss her terribly, but her unconditional love and her willingness to listen provided a stability that helped me get through eighth grade, high school and far beyond.

Unhappy Days

Even with Miss Simpson's support, high school was a brutal place. With no Catholic high schools in Woodland, many of my grammar school friends had gone on to Catholic high school in Sacramento. My father had considered sending me to Sacramento, but didn't want the hassle of the commute or car-pooling with other parents. Besides, my parents were not as committed to Catholicism as the commuters. My father had been raised Catholic but practiced his own form of Catholicism. This meant missing Sunday Mass occasionally or going to Mass late and leaving early. My mother had converted to Catholicism to marry my father. Though her church attendance was sporadic, she had a strong belief in God, the power of prayer, and the possibility of miracles.

During the first few weeks of public high school, my remaining eighth grade classmates from Catholic school and I stood at attention every time we were called on to answer a question. Sometimes we automatically answered, "Yes, Sister" or "No, Sister." The public school kids roared with laughter. Now that uniforms were no longer required, fashion mattered and I had to think about what outfit to wear and whether it would meet the dress code set by the ruling cliques. Any girl who wore the same dress two days in a row or who wore something "different" was considered a freak and an outcast. At least in grammar school, the dress code and social rules were well-defined. In high school, the rules were learned through observation or ostracism.

In the 1950s, only the real losers rode bikes to high school. Somehow, that was the cultural dictate. So I put aside my beloved Schwinn and walked the six blocks to school, sometimes crying all the way. I felt like I was back in kindergarten being dragged up the stairs while clinging to my mother. I was about to be fourteen, not five, but the same oppressive feelings of fear and sadness overwhelmed me. The simplest things–like changing classes every fifty minutes—upset me. I didn't like the hassle of changing clothes in P.E. and the need for two lockers, one in P.E. and the other along the corridor of classrooms. I became obsessed with remembering my locker codes, getting from class to class on time and having the right books. The only good thing about changing classes was being able to escape a disagreeable teacher or an annoying classroom of kids.

The worst part of the school day was lunchtime. Unlike grammar school, no one brought their lunch in a lunchbox. Wearing the wrong clothes, riding a bike, or eating from a lunchbox guaranteed instant freak status. There were only three ways to eat lunch: bring food in a brown paper bag, buy food from the cafeteria, or buy a hot dog or grilled cheese sandwich from an outside snack shack which the school operated during good weather. Buying from the cafeteria line meant you had to eat in the large cafeteria. This was great for the established cliques who occupied the same tables daily. The kids who didn't fit into specific groups either ate alone or joined other non-conversational loners. If I ate in the cafeteria, I was lucky to be able to sit with a good friend from grammar school. My favorite thing was to buy a grilled cheese sandwich and sit alone in the sun, but many times I was so close to tears I couldn't swallow my food. When this happened, I went into my empty fifth period classroom and started my homework.

Throughout my freshman year, I felt so shy and self-conscious that I wanted to evaporate. Ironically, my shyness made me feel even more conspicuous. I felt that my classmates could look inside me and view the unfolding of one of our ugly dinner scenes. Though being home was as stressful as being in school, I lived for the end of the school day. As I walked home, I wondered whether my mother would be out grocery shopping or home sober, drunk or somewhere in between.

I remember coming home from school one day and finding my mom collapsed in despair at the kitchen table. She lifted her head and said, "I just don't know what to do about your father. He treats me so badly. I'm so frightened all the time. I know I should stop drinking but I can't. I get so depressed I wish I were dead. I think you'd all be better off if I were dead. What do you think I should do? I rely on you to help me. You're the only person I can talk to."

"Mom, I tell you the same thing over and over. Why don't you get some kind of help? Go to a marriage counselor or get a divorce."

"I can't get a divorce. I'm a Catholic. Your father would never go to a marriage counselor because he thinks he's perfect. Everything is my fault."

"Well, I get tired of listening to these same problems. If you're not going to take my advice, why do you keep asking me to help you? All I hear about are the problems between you and dad. Nobody cares about my problems."

I listened to some version of my mother's complaints almost daily. After school, I tried to sneak into the house and into my bedroom before she saw me. But then I felt guilty for leaving her alone in her misery.

During my freshman year my father decided to change careers: He sold his retail store to become an insurance salesman. This change terrified my mother. She had liked the predictability of the retail hours, the consistency of my father's whereabouts and the ability to reach him by phone. Now my father had more freedom. He was happier and made more money. My mother hated his erratic work hours and evening appointments, during which she was unable to contact him. She became terrified of staying home without him on these evenings. As her obsession about his work hours turned to panic, her drinking increased and my father stayed away more evenings. I was left to watch her and my siblings.

I was trying to survive high school while worrying about my mother. One day after school, I found her passed out on her bedroom floor lying in a pool of vomit. I cleaned up the mess and dragged her into bed. She didn't wake up until I left for school the next morning. After this, I dreaded going home. Actually, I dreaded everything except the end of my freshman year.

I spent that summer trying to avoid my parents. I was sick of them and their problems. I locked myself in my bedroom and listened to the radio while I drew mandalas and worked with chalk and watercolors. I also spent hours on the tennis court making new friends and discovering how much anger and anxiety could be expelled by smacking a tennis ball. Occasionally, my mother and I played tennis. She was a natural athlete and had learned to play from her father, who had been a state tennis champion. During the times we played together, we had fun and our lives took on the feeling and appearance of an elusive normalcy.

Friends, Fitness and Facelifts

I started my sophomore year determined to make new friends. I joined the California Scholarship Federation, a scholastic achievement club. I shared classes with some sophomore members of the club and we began calling each other in the evenings to discuss homework. These were the students who became my friends for the remainder of high school.

It boosted my self-confidence to know that I fit into some slot of the high school pecking order. Inspired by my burgeoning confidence, I joined the Spanish Club and the Girls' Athletic Club. As a GAA member I could stay after school to play sports, thereby delaying the dreaded trip home. With sports and scholarship, I found my way into a relevant social group and into a seat at our own cafeteria table.

Now that I had friends, they wanted to come over after school and on weekends. In light of my mother's unpredictable drinking, the thought of having friends to the house terrified me. Instead, I went to their homes after school. On weekends I went to the movies with a group of girls or my new boyfriend, Tom.

In the spring of my sophomore year, my mother, inspired by Jack LaLanne, decided to get healthy. She went for long periods without drinking and developed an exercise routine. Her workout included jumping rope on the back patio in her underwear, swimming laps and lifting weights. She subscribed to bodybuilder magazines, which she hid from my father. She put Vaseline over her body to keep her skin from drying out and aging. A Vaseline oil slick floated on top of the pool water. The furniture and bed sheets became dark from the Vaseline. My mother lost track of time while exercising, which made for some late mealtimes.

At least now I thought it safe to bring my friends home. The only precaution I had to take was to make sure that my mother wasn't skipping rope in her underwear on the patio. When my friends met my mother, they loved her. When sober, she was witty, talkative and youthful. On many Saturday nights, my mother and I, my friends and my siblings and their friends sat around the kitchen table, talking and laughing past midnight. This was the mother I wanted permanently. But nothing remained stable or predictable in our house.

My mother had always been a person of extremes. For example, if one multivitamin was good for you, three were better. If thirty minutes of exercise was good, ninety would be ideal. She had gone from being a hypochondriac to a health nut and from drunkenness to abstinence.

Now at age 40 she began obsessing over her looks. She was beautiful in the classic manner of a Greta Garbo or Ingrid Bergman. She had been courted by a handsome, wealthy heir who had introduced her to a Hollywood agent interested in offering her a contract. From early on, she knew that her looks and brains were her most important assets, but money and stardom didn't appeal to her. Having survived a tumultuous and unstable childhood, she craved the stability and normalcy she saw in my father's closely knit Italian family. Dazzled by her beauty, my father had pursued her relentlessly. Once when I asked my mother why she married him she replied, "He wouldn't leave me alone. I couldn't get rid of him. Whenever I went out my front door, I had to step over him."

When my mother started obsessing on her looks, she wouldn't stop talking about it. "I don't want to get flabby and wrinkled. That's why I exercise and use Vaseline." She'd look at her face from every angle in the mirror. "I really need a facelift. Maybe one of my brothers will give me the money. If not, I'll have to save up for it out of the grocery money. I'm going to find the best plastic surgeon in the area and get an opinion." She consulted with a plastic surgeon who told her to return in five years; she didn't need surgery now and would be wasting her money.

After that news, she developed a "do-it-yourself" strategy. This involved pulling her hair away from her face at night and taping the loose skin by her eyes and mouth tightly to the skin at the edge of her face. After the taping, she put Vaseline over her face and body. When my father saw her like this he'd strut around the house saying, "I can't believe what I'm seeing. Nobody in their right mind would want to go to bed every night with you. You look like a goddam mummy. Your looks are more important than anything else. Well, I'm over your looks. I just want to be with a normal woman who cooks and cleans house." My father began working longer hours and my mother went into funks over her midlife face. She started drinking again, but not as often or as much as before her fitness obsession.

Besta

When my maternal grandmother came to live with us she was sixty-nine. We had always called her Besta, for Bestamore, which means grandmother in Norwegian. She was the daughter of Norwegian immigrants who settled in Wisconsin. As Besta matured, she showed no interest in staying on the Wisconsin farm and marrying a farmer; she wanted to go to college. She was granted a full scholarship to Valparaiso University in Indiana, graduating in the early 1900s as valedictorian. She married a brilliant metallurgical engineer who had graduated from college in his mid-teens. He had family ties to well-known politicians and newspaper moguls. My mother told me the two of them could have done great things together, but their lives were ruined by my grandfather's alcoholism.

After years of financial and emotional turmoil, Besta took her three young children and left her husband. She struggled to raise her children by herself and was forced to move often to find work. Eventually, she settled in San

Francisco where she worked selling a motley assortment of products including encyclopedias and real estate. Heroically, her three children, my mother and two brothers, also worked to keep food on the table and eviction notices off the door.

Besta was unlike my paternal grandmother or any other grandmother I knew. She was tall and thin, with perfect posture and a stately bearing. Her perfectly coiffed silver-blue hair contrasted nicely with the navy business suit she wore whenever we visited her in San Francisco. She was well-read and knowledgeable and talked for hours about everything. Before she moved in with us, she had visited us often and encouraged us to read and learn by bringing each of us an inscribed book with every visit. My siblings and I looked forward to her visits because she read to us every night and rubbed our backs before tucking us in. She helped us with our homework and when I was stuck on an algebra problem, she could solve it in her head. This always amazed me!

But the Besta who moved in with us my junior year was no longer the same person who could solve math problems in her head. Every morning when I got up for school, Besta was already up fumbling around the kitchen. She tried to help us out by putting cereal bowls on the table, but when we went to the cupboard containing the cereal and sugar, they were missing. When opening the refrigerator to get the milk, either the sugar or cereal would be there. I started getting up earlier just so I could find breakfast. Sometimes the cereal box would be in the unheated oven, the sugar bowl would be tucked away in a drawer or the milk would be in a cupboard. If I asked Besta where anything was, she'd look at me blankly. After finding stove burners left on or pans with no food left on burners, my mother knew she couldn't leave Besta home alone. In order to run errands my mother either took Besta with her or waited until I came home from school to watch her. It felt strange to be watching over the grandmother who used to watch over me.

My father, who had always found Besta annoying and opinionated, would get up extra early in the mornings to avoid her. He avoided being in the same room with her as much as possible. At dinner, he would bolt his food and leave for an appointment. He never offered to help my mother with anything. His lack of help and compassion toward my mother hurt her feelings and made her angry and dependent on me. Besta, who was not totally incapacitated, understood that my father avoided her and that her presence might be creating problems. My mother, caught between placating my father and caring for her mother, became severely depressed and anxious. I could tell that much of the time she was on the verge of tears and I hoped she could continue to keep her drinking to a minimum. Now when she drank, she seemed capable of maintaining a comfortable plateau. Still I worried about the tenuous state of her sobriety and wondered what event or level of stress might push her over the edge.

When my mother finally took Besta to the doctor, he diagnosed her with "senile dementia" due to hardening of the arteries. He claimed that dementia was a normal part of aging, which we now know is not always true. The incorrect diagnosis couldn't be blamed on the doctor. In the 1950s, Alzheimer's disease was unknown to both doctors and the public. Though in 1906, Dr. Alois Alzheimer had seen the plaques and tangles in the brain of one of his patients, it wasn't until the 1970s, after years of skepticism and research, that Alzheimer's disease became recognized as a separate disease, not a normal part of aging.

During my junior year I got my long-awaited driver's license. I loved cars and I loved to drive. My father had his own car, his precious trophy Cadillac which nobody else was allowed to drive. Our second car, which my mother and I drove, was always a Chevy or Buick convertible. There was nothing more freeing than putting the top down and driving away from our house. I lived for Friday and Saturday nights when my friends and I piled into the convertible and cruised.

Late one night in spring while driving down Main Street, I sideswiped a parked car. It was after midnight and nobody was around. I panicked. Without realizing that I should have left a note on the other car's windshield, I drove home. Luckily, my mother was still up and my father was asleep. When I told my mother what I had done, she came undone. She and I went into the garage to assess the damage. There was about a two-inch wide and four-foot long area on the right side of the car where the white paint was scraped away, showing the gray undercoat. My mother was frantic. "I have to fix this before your father sees it. If he sees it, he'll have a fit and blame me. I just can't take any more problems. Life's hard enough with him complaining about my mother living here." She looked around wildly. "I think there's some white house paint and paint brushes in the garage. I'll cover the scrape with the house paint and hope he doesn't notice. You must never tell him what happened."

I said, "But mom, it was just an accident. Everyone has accidents."

"With your father, nothing is just an accident. An accident to your father is an excuse to blame someone, usually me, for being incompetent."

I couldn't believe she was going to paint the car with house paint. As I watched her paint, I noticed that her hands were shaking and she was about to cry. I felt the all too familiar lump in my throat and the heaviness in my heart. I wanted to do something to help her, to make her feel better, but it was impossible. I kept wishing that she'd quit being so terrified of my father. I couldn't understand why she didn't stand up to him. What was she afraid of? Being left alone? Feeling abandoned like she did in childhood by an alcoholic father or by moving frequently and getting stuck in boarding schools? My mother was smart. Why couldn't she use her brains to overpower my father? Many of my friends' mothers bossed their husbands around. Why couldn't my mother do it? These were questions I pondered frequently.

Now my mother obsessed on the effectiveness of her paint job. Every day that passed without my father noticing the patched area on the car, my mother was relieved. When weeks of obsessive worry passed without my father saying a word about the car, my mother let go of the incident.

As the summer after my junior year approached, my father started nagging me about getting a job. He suggested that I teach swimming in our pool. At first I was skeptical about the idea. Just because I was a good swimmer didn't mean I could be a good teacher. I had to learn how to teach what I knew. I discovered from the city recreation department that the Red Cross gave lessons in lifesaving and teaching swimming. I signed up for the first classes in June. With my teaching certification and lifesaving badge in hand, I put an ad in the paper. I had enough responses to stay booked all summer. Teaching swimming proved to be a gratifying and lucrative job. Not only did I teach, but I learned. I learned I could exercise some control over my life and that I could overcome some of my torturous shyness.

That same summer, I learned something I didn't want to know: that my father was capable of hitting my mother. It happened one summer evening when my father was hosting a dinner party for his coworkers and some high-ranking executives from the insurance company. My father had been looking forward to the party for weeks. The backyard was perfectly planted and manicured, the Japanese lanterns were strung across the yard and the table and chairs were meticulously arranged. The night of the dinner, the men arrived in suits and ties while the women wore elegant summer dresses. This was to be the perfect evening. My father, a top producer in the company, considered it an honor to be entertaining the executives. My mother, looking gorgeous in a purple silk dress, was the designated cook, hostess and waitress.

The night of the party, I parked on the living room couch so I could watch everyone. I was worried about my mother and her ability to stay sober during the party. She had been stressed and depressed over her mother's illness and my father's ongoing disapproval of Besta's presence. Considering what my mother was dealing with, I thought my father's expectations for her to perform flawlessly for the benefit of his ego were unreasonable.

I cringed when I saw my mother sipping from the bourbon bottle under the sink. With each tray of hors d'oeuvres or dinner that she carried to the table, her walk became more unsteady. Noticing this, my father excused himself, grabbed my mother by the hand and brought her into the living room. He threw her down onto the couch and started screaming at her, "You're drunk again and you're ruining my party. Why did you have to get drunk tonight? You're embarrassing me in front of the people I work with. I won't stand for this. Pull yourself together and get back outside."

My mother sobbed. "I can't go back out there. I can't take anymore. I need to go to bed."

With no warning, my father slapped her across the face so hard that it left a red handprint.

She cried even more. "How could you do this to me? Can't you see I'm coming apart? I need help."

Viciously, he said, "You don't need help. You just need to quit drinking. You're a no-good drunk and you've made a mess of the evening."

Trembling, I yelled at my father, "How dare you hit mom! What kind of a man hits his wife? Go away and leave her alone." It felt good to scream at him. I knew it was safe to confront him because he had to get back to the guests. When he was back outside, my mother went into her bedroom. He told the company that his wife was ill and lying down. "Hopefully, she'll join us later." My mother returned in time to get the dessert on the table and help clean up the dishes.

As of that night, my mother's drinking was no longer a secret; too many people were paying attention and had watched her stagger with the dinner trays. The fight between my parents over the events of that evening raged on for days. I felt sorry for Besta who was confused by it all, perhaps thinking that her presence was to blame. As my parents fought, my mother admitted that she was an alcoholic who couldn't stop drinking on her own. She needed help. Help and sobriety did arrive later, but in the meantime, chaos prevailed.

Overwhelmed

By the fall of 1959, the start of my senior year, Besta had been living with us for a year. My father, who had been growing increasingly intolerant of her presence, insisted that she had to leave. The idea of having to relocate Besta caused my mother great anguish. Besta had spent most of her life moving from place to place. She had never owned a home. My mother wanted to give her a secure and comfortable place to live for the years that remained before her dementia deprived her of all sense of time and place.

As my mother pondered what to do with Besta and the cruelty of her eviction, she sank into a dark depression. Over the years, I had watched my mother flow in and out of many depressions, but the idea of abandoning Besta threw her into a new low. She called her older brother in Alaska for advice. He suggested that Besta move in with his family until a more permanent solution could be found. Since Besta had been to Alaska many times to visit her son, my mother and her brother agreed that the temporary move would not startle her. When Besta left for Anchorage, my mother missed her but found relief from my father's complaining. Life seemed strange without Besta padding around the house, trying to be helpful. Her departure was the first of many unpleasant events that would unfold during my senior year.

That fall, the college-prep seniors began sending applications to the colleges they wanted to attend. My father had already decided I was going to attend the University of California, Davis, located twelve miles from home. One day after class, my art teacher, Mr. Reilly, asked me to meet with him after school to talk about college. He recommended that I attend a private Catholic college in San Diego operated by the Madames of the Sacred Heart, a prestigious teaching community of Catholic nuns. One of the art teachers at the college was Sister Corita Kent, famous for her serigraphs, which combined words, color and shapes. In the sixties and seventies, posters of her work could be found hanging in schools, dorm rooms and in print ads. Since my artwork was abstract and geometric, he thought she would be the perfect mentor for me, someone who could launch me into a career in painting and graphic design.

I owned several of Sister Kent's posters and books. I was thrilled about the possibility of learning from her. When I told Mr. Reilly that my father had plans for me to go to UC Davis, he said, "I'll come to your house and talk to your father. I believe so strongly in your talent and ability to make it in the art world, I'd do anything to get you to the right instructor. Studying with Corita Kent would be perfect for you and would give you the opportunity of a lifetime." What a surprise that my teacher thought highly enough of my ability to challenge my father!

Mr. Reilly arrived early on a Saturday morning. My mother was still in bed but my father and I were sitting in the living room. After polite introductions, Mr. Reilly stated his case.

"Your daughter is a talented artist with great potential. She has been one of my best students for four years. She loves art and I recommend that she attend a private Catholic college in San Diego where she can study with a renowned graphic artist who would be a good fit for her."

My father launched into one of his diatribes. "I've already signed Diane up for UCD. I want my kids to go to a UC school. I graduated from UC Berkeley and those years were the best of my life. If UC was good enough for me, it's good enough for my kids. Besides, artists don't make any money, and my daughter needs to make a living. She needs to be a teacher. The Catholic college is a private school and would cost a fortune. UCD is close to home and she could commute if necessary. Besides, her mother would have a fit if her daughter went far away to school. You have no right coming over here to tell me what's best for my kids."

Mr. Reilly, a gentle and caring man, looked shocked when my father escorted him to the door and slammed it behind him. I screamed at my father, "You have no idea who I am or what's best for me. You're trying to control my life and I'm sick of it. There's no excuse for the way you treated Mr. Reilly, someone who understands me and is trying to help. No wonder everyone thinks you're an asshole!"

I ran into my room and slammed and locked the door. He ran after me yelling, "What did you call me? How dare you talk to me like that! I should beat the living daylights out of you. Open that door now." He was like a rabid dog, snarling and snapping there on the other side of the door.

I thought about climbing out my bedroom window and walking to a friend's house until my father cooled off. But this strategy had backfired in the past. I eventually had to come home and when I did, he was twice as mad.

The commotion brought my mother out of her bedroom. When I heard her coming down the hall, I left my bedroom and followed her into the living room. My father would be too busy with her to continue attacking me. My mother was confused by the commotion. "What's going on here? Who was at the door?"

My father replied, "It was the art teacher from high school. He came over to tell me about a college in San Diego where we should send Diane. He was going on about developing her artistic talent but I set him straight. I told him she was going to UCD and that I made the decisions about my kids."

The only two words my mother seemed to hear were San Diego. This freaked her out and she started crying. "San Diego! She can't go to San Diego. It's too far from home. I couldn't survive with her that far away." My mother kept sobbing. "I can't take any more fighting and problems. I just don't want to be here any longer. I'm going back to my room to lie down."

My father told her, "Quit exaggerating everything and quit feeling sorry for yourself. The only person you care about is yourself and whether you'll be left alone."

The house grew quiet as my mother shuffled off to the bathroom where I could hear her rummaging around the medicine cabinet. Then I heard the rattle of pills being shaken out of a bottle. My father and I were still sitting in the living room and as soon as she was out of sight, I asked him if we should check on her. "What if she kills herself?"

Then he started on a tirade. "This is the kind of shit I put up with all the time. She's always threatening to kill herself just to get attention or manipulate people. She can't stand the thought of her kids leaving home or going too far away. She's never wanted to be alone. When you kids were small, I had to bring her to the store with me because she couldn't stay home without me. If you were to go far away to school and your mother killed herself, it would be your fault. Think about that."

I did just that. I sat there angry and hurt, thinking about what kind of father would say something so horrific to one of his children! What kind of father would put that kind of burden on his child?

While I was still thinking about what he had just said, he continued to talk. "I don't think I ever told you about your mother trying to kill herself when she was pregnant with you. Your mother was always vain. She was obsessed with her looks and body. When she realized that being pregnant would give her stretch marks, she was horrified. When she was a few months pregnant with you, I found her sitting in the car with a hose hooked up, the garage door shut and the engine on. She was awake when I got her out of the car. When I asked her what the hell she was doing, she said that she didn't want to be pregnant because it would ruin her body. I knew then that I never should have married her. I've stuck it out all these years for you kids."

I was dumbfounded by this revelation. I couldn't believe he was telling me this. Incapable of absorbing the information, I doubted its credibility. Was he telling me the truth? My mother was vain, but did she really try to kill herself when she was pregnant? Why was he unloading this on me? Was it to keep me close to home and make me forever responsible for my mother?

While I remained speechless, pondering his revelations, I remembered hearing my mother shake out pills from a bottle and wondering if and what she had ingested. My father followed me into the bedroom to discover she had taken half a bottle of aspirin. She was asleep. My father assured me she'd be fine and we left her alone.

She was fine but I wasn't. I agonized over the startling revelation of my mother's early suicide attempt. I dreaded going to UCD in the fall and I was too embarrassed to go back to art class. The Monday following Mr. Reilly's visit, I went to him after class and said, "I want to apologize for my father's rudeness. Thanks for taking the time to come over and for believing in my talent. I wish my parents felt the same way."

He said, "It's not your responsibility to apologize for your father. I wish I could have been more helpful. Just remember that whatever happens in the future, you have a talent that will always be part of you. Nobody can ever take that away from you."

Surgery

In early spring of 1960, my uncle brought Besta back to our house. He was a contractor and real estate developer who took the Alaskan winters off. His work began again in spring and he could no longer watch over Besta. Once again, my mother was faced with the question of what to do with her mother. My father had made it clear that she couldn't move back in with us permanently; she could only stay until my mother could find a place for her. He wanted my mother to start looking immediately. In the sixties, few long-term care facilities existed. The two in town were for critically ill or severely demented patients. Besta was still ambulatory and capable of some speech and understanding. The only place my mother could find was a less-than-desirable rooming house for the elderly located on Main Street, not far from our house. After discussing the cost of the facility with her brothers, my mother signed Besta up for the boarding house.

On the morning of Besta's move-in day, I was in school and my father was working. My mother took Besta by herself. When I got home from school, I found my mother sitting at the kitchen table sobbing. I asked, "Mom, why are you crying?"

"It was so hard for me to take my mother to that boarding house today. The place is so depressing I felt like I was dumping mom in hell. I just can't fathom why I have to leave her in some strange place when we live just a few blocks away."

"How did Besta do with the move?"

"She seemed sad and confused but she didn't complain. You know how she is; she is stoic. She never asks for anything or complains about anything. She's had a hard life and knows that complaining doesn't change things. Besides, she prides herself on being a strong, stoic Scandinavian. I just feel so badly for her. At least I can visit her every day, but it will be so terribly hard to leave her behind. I'll bring her to the house for regular visits and for the holidays, but it will be heartbreaking to have to take her back to the boarding house." I felt so sad for my mother and Besta.

My mother visited Besta almost daily, and even this annoyed my father. He expected her primary focus to be tending to his priorities of cleaning, cooking and entertaining. He never asked about Besta or accompanied my mother when she visited. His lack of interest and moral support added to her sadness, anxiety and depression. Her only comfort resided in a bourbon bottle.

My mother was like a doormat. I wanted to shake her until she woke up and stood up to my father. Instead, I dwelled on my own problems and my immediate post-high school future, headed for a university I didn't want to attend. Though I wanted to get away from my parents, I felt the magnetic pull of my mother's neediness.

In May of 1960, a month before high school graduation, I experienced two days of constant, intense abdominal pain. My mother convinced my reluctant father that I needed to see a doctor. She took me to the hospital. After a day of pelvic exams and blood work, the doctors had no diagnosis. By mid-afternoon, my white cell count had risen, my blood pressure had dropped and my pulse rate had increased. Thinking that I might have appendicitis and was going into shock, the doctors decided to operate.

As I was being prepared for surgery, my mother was presented with a consent form. For financial reasons, she was afraid to sign the form without my father's permission. She called everywhere looking for him and leaving messages for him to call the hospital. He came racing in about 4:00 p.m. to assess the situation.

The surgeon and my parents were talking outside the door of my hospital room. My mother understood why I needed surgery but my father wanted an explanation. The doctor started with "Your daughter's pain and vital signs are worrisome and I'm afraid if we don't operate soon, she'll go into shock and we could lose her in the operating room. We can't give an exact diagnosis until we get inside. The most likely cause for her symptoms is appendicitis but it could be something else. If it were my daughter, she would have been in surgery two hours ago."

My father responded, "What do you mean you don't know what's wrong with her? Why would you operate on someone when you don't know what's wrong? How much is this going to cost me? I need to know the cost before I'll sign the form. If you operate and find nothing, then I'm out a lot of money."

I was lying in bed listening to this unbelievable dialogue. I could tell from the doctor's tone of voice that he was exasperated and angry. He said, "Look, sir. Your daughter may die without surgery. In fact, we're losing precious time arguing about this. I can't give you an exact price for the operation. It depends on what we find in surgery and the length of her hospital stay. I don't believe you can put a price tag on a life. How will you feel if we can't stabilize her and she dies in surgery?"

On hearing this, I panicked. I hadn't given much thought to death until now. I just wanted my father to sign the forms and get this resolved. My life was fading while he was being obstinate. The instant he finally signed, I was wheeled through two sets of large doors leading to the operating room. A small, spiteful part of me hoped I would never come out. I pictured my death haunting and punishing my father for the rest of his days. As I listened to the operating room staff talking to each other, I realized that a larger, more rational part of me wanted to live and I trusted the doctor to make that happen.

The operation revealed that my left ovary had ruptured during ovulation and bled out into my abdomen. The surgeon mended the torn ovary and removed several pints of blood that had filled the abdominal cavity. Later, he explained that anytime blood is not where it is supposed to be in the body, it causes severe pain and can lead to shock. He was amazed I had survived walking to school for two days during which time I was undoubtedly bleeding internally.

I stayed in the hospital stitched and bandaged for two miserable weeks of pain and itching. I recuperated in time to take final exams and to march weakly through the graduation ceremony.

To avoid thinking about my mother's steady decline and my fear of going to UC Davis, I focused on having fun during my senior summer. When I wasn't teaching swimming, I hung out with my high school friends. We played tennis, swam until midnight, rode horseback, cruised Main Street, played records, went to the movies and the county fair. We all felt that this would be our last summer together and we had to make the most of it.

Though Tom and I dated almost every weekend during school, we saw each other sporadically over the summer. He had gone to Tahoe to work at a general store in Tahoe City as he had every summer during high school. He lived at his parents' vacation home not far from his job. We were able to date when I went to Tahoe with my parents or when he drove to Woodland on his days off. When apart, he wrote long, romantic letters to me daily. Tom was special to me. He was handsome, personable, smart, romantic and ambitious. We believed we were deeply in love and that we had a future together. But neither of us wanted to make promises that time and distance might erode. I was going to UC Davis and he was headed for UC Santa Barbara, six hours south of Davis. His goal was to become a doctor, a goal I never doubted he would achieve.

By the end of August, my friends and Tom were getting ready to head out of town for college. The summer fun was over and I felt lonely and abandoned. Besta was slowly deteriorating and my mother was dealing with the pain by drinking more. Actually, my mother was rolling downhill faster than Besta and my normally obtuse father started to take notice. He now realized that telling my mother to stop drinking was useless. Finally understanding she needed help, he contacted an old friend, Harvey, a recovering alcoholic who attended AA meetings regularly. Harvey agreed to come over and talk with my mother about his experience with AA. When he arrived with some AA material, my mother listened with great skepticism but agreed to attend a meeting with him. She made it through three meetings with Harvey, then quit.

One day in August, my mother and I were in the bathroom together. She was looking at herself in the mirror and not liking what she saw. She said, "I really look terrible. I know if I don't stop drinking, I'm going to die. I'm just so frightened all the time I don't know how I can face life sober. I know that my drinking has taken a terrible toll on you kids and I'm sorry for that. Maybe if I can change, your father might change. I pray every night that I'll find my way to some place where I can get the right kind of help."

I went into my room and sobbed.

A Sober Mother

In late August of 1960, my mother drove me the twelve miles to UC Davis. As she helped me put away my clothes in my assigned dorm room, she talked to me like I was moving to New York. "I'm going to miss you so much. I'll call you every day to see how you're doing. Things just won't be the same without you. I'll come get you every weekend so you can spend the weekends at home." I felt like a freak having a clingy, semi-drunk mother who showed up on Fridays to take me home. On the weekends I didn't go home, I felt guilty. My mother needed me for company and to accompany her to visit Besta.

The road she took to the university was a busy two-lane highway with large walnut trees bordering each side. One Friday when she arrived at school, I could tell she'd been drinking heavily. I got into the passenger side and let her drive. When we got onto the highway, my mother began weaving all over the road. I was terrified. When she crossed over the yellow line, oncoming cars honked and swerved out of the way. I said, "Mom, you're weaving all over the road. You're going to kill us or somebody else."

She slurred out the words, "No I'm not. I'm fine. You worry too much." She was oblivious to the danger she posed. We made it home, but I insisted on driving every time we were together and worried about her driving by herself. I knew I should tell my father but was afraid he'd forbid her to drive, which might cause her to drink even more. The problem took care of itself one afternoon in late September when she ran off the side of the road and hit a tree. Luckily, nobody was hurt. It happened right outside of town where someone who knew her gave her a ride home. The car had minor damage but had to be towed out of a small ditch to the repair shop. My mother was already home when the police came with a damage report for the insurance company. Since nobody else was involved, she wasn't cited. The combination of my father's fury and the accident scared her into looking for a rehabilitation facility.

She found an article in the *San Francisco Chronicle* about an alcohol rehab clinic in Redwood City, which claimed a high rate of treatment success. She called and signed herself up for the three-week program. She left home the first week in October, the week I turned eighteen.

The day my mother left, the weather was terrible. The thought of driving to Redwood City frightened her. The city is located about 110 miles from our home and about twenty-five miles south of San Francisco. To get there, she'd have to drive in heavy traffic and cross the Bay Bridge. Because driving on busy freeways and in big cities made her nervous, she asked my father to take her. My father refused. He told her it was her problem and it was up to her to fix it. Instead of being glad that she wanted to stop drinking, he punished her by forcing her to drive alone in a compromised state. I worried about whether she'd make it to the facility alive. I admired her courage and strength and imagined her driving through that rainstorm with her hands shaking on the steering wheel.

While my mother was in rehab, she wrote to me daily. The clinic practiced aversion therapy, which has been used to treat alcoholism since the early 1930s. She described this method of treatment in one of her letters. "Tomorrow I receive another treatment. It is quite miserable, which is the entire object. They inject something into you and pour enormous quantities of salt water and all types of booze into you and you become incredibly sick. After the treatments, you associate alcohol with this dreadful response and you don't want to touch another drop." She stuck it out for the prescribed three weeks. When she completed the program, she drove herself home.

When my mother returned from the clinic, I presumed that my parents would interact differently. I hoped that my father would stop verbally abusing her and that she would stop putting up with his attacks. My mother expressed her concerns in a letter to me.

"At the clinic, they warned me how very difficult it would be for me to follow their program if I had to come home to such threatening, nagging and hammering. However, I will make it anyway." She continues, "I am trying so very hard it is really too bad that he is so unwilling to put forth any effort. Perhaps if I can succeed, he will somehow change. Having used alcohol as a crutch to deaden my sensibilities against problems and his incessant pounding, it is very hard at first to adjust to standing without a leaning post."

Neither of my parents' behavior changed immediately. Eventually, with no alcohol to fuel her feelings of low self-esteem, my mother became emotionally stronger and more assertive. She began to see that when she stood up for herself, my father backed down.

During the remainder of my freshman year, my mother still came to visit but not as often. When I did go home for a weekend, I accompanied her to see Besta who had broken a hip and now resided in the gruesome geriatric ward of the hospital where everyone looked the same: sitting in wheelchairs with their heads down. Sometimes, my mother and I would have to bend over patients' faces to find Besta. My mother cried every time she left the hospital. I cried when I looked into peoples' faces looking for Besta. So many times my mother said, "I wish I didn't have to go through this sober. It would be so easy for me to start drinking again. It takes all the willpower I can muster to see mom like this and stay sober." While she mustered her willpower, I remained vigilant for any signs of relapse.

My Junior Year

My junior year at Davis was filled with change and surprise. Tom and I had drifted apart and were no longer dating. He was involved with his pre-med studies and his duties as president of his fraternity. Life at home had improved. My mother hadn't relapsed and my parents seemed happier. My dorm roommate, Susan, and I moved into an off-campus apartment. We were tired of dorm food and dorm rules, which included boring, mandatory meetings. Though apartment living offered more freedom, on-campus living offered the ease of getting around by foot or bicycle and a place to return to between classes. With the move, I had to bike several miles to class and spend hours in the library between long class breaks. Susan had a car, which was no help to me because our class times and days differed dramatically. So while she drove to school when it rained, I rode my bike, only to arrive soaked and irritated.

After suffering through several colds, fevers, and tonsillitis, which had negatively affected my studies and attendance, I begged my father for a car. I was worn out and about to quit school when he bought me a low-end Chevy sedan. He bought it on the condition that I pay for gas and upkeep, as he was footing all my other bills. To support a car, I needed a job.

I took a part-time job at the local newspaper which was owned by the Sloans, a couple from Woodland who owned newspapers in Davis and Woodland. I quickly learned that the newspaper people I worked with were a different breed. They were an independent, eccentric group who chain-smoked and lived on coffee and junk-food. When Mrs. Sloan visited the Davis office, she frequently left her car double-parked for long periods of time with the engine running. She was not being defiant; she was just scatterbrained. The police, who were tired of threatening to tow her car, just let it sit idling in the street while everyone drove around it. In addition to double-parking, she was prone to leaving the gas station without paying. The station owner would periodically show up at the paper with a stack of receipts to be paid from the petty cash drawer. Mrs. Sloan wore thick, black-framed glasses, black and white dresses, and over-sized, white high-heels that sounded like horses' hooves. She looked like Minnie Mouse.

Though I was hired as a proofreader, I quickly learned to do many things. I worked in the classified ad department, helped with page layout, subscriptions and billing. Every time I started to proofread, I got called away to do something else. The more I learned, the more work I was given and I often stayed long after my shift ended. When deadlines loomed and the pressure mounted, the employees fought with each other and everyone fought with the editor. I loved working there amidst the daily crises and chaos. I was comfortable there—it felt like home.

When spring of 1963 arrived with its usual beautiful weather, I dreamed of owning a sports car. I laid awake nights figuring out how to come up with enough money to buy a Jaguar. On one of my free days, I drove to the Jaguar dealership in Sacramento to get an idea of price and to gaze at the beautiful inventory. I made several trips there before I got up the nerve to talk to a salesman, who was astounded that I was shopping for myself. I couldn't afford a new car but the salesman showed me a used 1961 XKE silver roadster that I fell in love with. The price was $5,200. When the salesman put the top down and took me for a drive, I knew I had to buy that Jaguar. I put $200 down to hold the car for a week while I came up with a plan.

Before I could approach my father, I needed a fully-formed financial plan. The salesman put together some figures for me to consider. The dealership would allow about $1,200 for the Chevy as a trade-in and I could contribute $1,000 from my savings. To make up the remainder, I'd have to get a loan from my father or a bank. The salesman had recommended a bank one block from the dealership that specialized in car loans. When I left the salesman, I walked to the bank and asked some surprised loan officer for financing. He took my request seriously and explained that I'd need a co-signer on the note. The idea of discussing this matter with my father terrified me, but my desire for the car was greater than my fear. What did I have to lose? If he said no, I still had the Chevy.

I picked a day when he was in a good mood and said, "Dad, I need to talk to you about something. I want to trade-in the Chevy for a sports car. I know this sounds crazy, but I've wanted a sports car since I got my driver's license. I've been to the Jaguar dealership and to the bank. I've got all the details."

My father was shocked. "You went shopping for a car and to the bank by yourself? You must me serious about this. But I just bought you a car a few months ago and it's paid for. Why would you want to be stuck making car payments? By the way, how are you going to make the payments and pay for the upkeep of a Jaguar? Those cars are gas guzzlers and they're expensive to work on."

I laid out my plan consisting of the Chevy trade-in, my $1,000, and the rest from the bank. "I'll be able to make the payments with my newspaper money. They want me to work full-time over the summer and part-time my senior year. After I graduate, I'll get a teaching job."

"All right," he said, running his hand through his hair. "I'll go to the dealership with you to see the car and the paperwork. If everything looks fine, we'll go to the bank. I'll co-sign for you with one understanding: If you miss a payment, don't come to me for the money. If I should loan you money for a payment, you must pay it back. You have to be totally responsible for the car. Do you understand?" He fixed me with a stern look.

"Yes, dad. I understand." I said, my heart leaping. "I'll do whatever it takes to pay for the car. Thanks for helping me!"

When my father saw the XKE, his jaw dropped. "This is a beautiful car! Maybe you'll let me drive it!"

After the transaction was completed, the salesman handed me the keys to the Jag. It was then I realized I had no idea how to drive the car. I'd driven an H-pattern column shift in driver education, but it bore no resemblance to the Jag's floor shift. The salesman went over the gear pattern and the use of the clutch, but to no avail. I drove the twelve miles to Woodland in second gear. After hours of grinding gears and jerking my way around quiet streets, I eventually mastered the art of smooth shifting.

I loved my car. I washed and waxed it regularly. Though it turned heads everywhere I went, the most thrilling part of driving the Jag was the feeling of freedom that came with the wind blowing my hair, the roar of the engine, and the power and speed that could be unleashed in seconds. Within those seconds, I moved further away from the restrictions and demands of school, work, and my mother.

Toward the end of my junior year, I met Dave. My father and Dave's parents had become friends after they had purchased a substantial amount of insurance from my dad. Dave's parents, who were meeting their son in Sacramento on a Friday night for dinner, invited my parents to join them. My father offered to bring me along to meet Dave, who was living in an apartment and attending Sacramento State, studying history. When my father called to tell me he'd arranged this meeting, it was on the Friday morning of the dinner and I was busy cramming for Monday's final exams. I was ill-prepared for my tests and in no mood to meet anyone. I was furious with my father. "How could you sign me up for a date without asking me? I have finals on Monday and I need to study. I'm not going. You can tell them I'm sick or whatever. Besides, I barely have enough time to get ready."

In his usual autocratic way, my father said, "I've already arranged this meeting and you're coming. These people are wealthy clients and you're not backing out. You can study over the weekend."

"But Dad-"

"Your mother and I will pick you up about four. We're going to Dave's apartment for appetizers and drinks, then out to dinner."

We rode to Sacramento in silence. When we arrived, I was introduced to Dave and his parents. After seeing Dave, I was glad I came. He was a few inches taller than my 5'4" and he looked like his handsome, Italian father. Both had brown hair and eyes, refined features and full lips. With his natty dress, polished demeanor and good looks, he reminded me of Robert Wagner. He took drink orders and passed around the hors d'oeuvres he had made. When it came time to head for the restaurant, Dave asked if I'd like to ride with him. Thrilled by the invitation, I was even more excited when I saw his car. He opened the passenger door and I got into a gorgeous, 1960 gold Corvette.

Our dinner destination was Frank Fat's, a landmark Chinese restaurant located in downtown Sacramento close to the capitol. It was famous for its strong drinks and the legislators who gathered there for lunch. My parents, who frequented the restaurant, knew the owner, the bartenders and the waiters. I had been going to Frank Fat's with my parents and their friends since I was small. On many weekend nights, I was lifted onto a bar stool where I could watch the bartenders mix drinks. When the bartenders weren't busy, they fussed over me and treated me to Shirley Temples.

The restaurant fascinated me. The bar was huge with mirrors and lights along the back wall that reflected and backlit the large and colorful inventory. I watched in awe as the bartenders mixed drinks with incredible speed. When I wasn't watching the bartenders, I looked around at the patrons and the decor. The gold, fire-breathing dragons, the Chinese scenes and lettering painted on the red walls made me feel like I had been transported to an exotic and mysterious land. On our trips home from Lake Tahoe, we frequently stopped at Frank Fat's for dinner. Though my patronage has waned over the years, I've held onto the good memories and my early fascination with a restaurant that had sparked my imagination.

When Dave and I, along with the parents, sat down at a bar table that Friday evening, I thought it auspicious that my first date with Dave was taking place in my old make-believe land of enchantment. As I sat there, I daydreamed about the past, sipped my beer and made small-talk with Dave. The parents, with the exception of my mother, were quickly going through rounds of bourbon drinks. I went to the bathroom and when I returned, a gin martini was sitting by my beer. I asked, "Where did this come from? I didn't order it and I don't want it."

Dave's mother grinned slyly, "I ordered it. I thought you might like a martini. Why don't you try it?"

I didn't want to be rude so I complied. I sipped the martini cautiously until it was gone. Since we had been drinking for over an hour, the martini made me dizzy and I told Dave I had to eat right away. As I sobered up with food, I wondered why Dave's mother had pushed the martini on me. It was a strange and confusing incident.

After dinner, Dave insisted on driving me back to Davis. On the way, we talked about how much we'd enjoyed ourselves. We discussed the food and ambience of Frank Fat's and my long history with the restaurant. I told him a silly story about my father and Frank Fat's. "One Sunday morning, after an evening at Fat's, I found my father lying on the living room floor. I asked him, "'What's the matter with you?'"

I laughed when he answered, "Oh, I have a dreadful hangover. It's that Chinese food. It makes me drunk."

After my father story, Dave and I moved to a discussion of our respective fathers, both of whom were sons of Italian immigrants. We talked about "the Italian thing"— the fussiness about food, the complaining, the neurotic perfectionism and the compulsive house-cleaning. We conversed so easily, I regretted the short trip to Davis. When we arrived, Dave walked me to my apartment door. He left with a promise to call.

Courtship and Marriage

When the semester ended, Dave and I moved back to our respective home towns for the summer. We had every intention of dating on weekends, but my job got in the way a lot. My days at the paper started at 9:00 a.m. and usually lasted until 10:00 at night. I was needed in both the Woodland and Davis locations and worked Monday through Friday as well as some Saturdays. I did my usual 9:00 to 5:00 stint in Davis, then rushed home to Woodland for dinner. After dinner, I proofread at the Woodland office. I worked in a small cubicle in the pressroom where the paper was printed. I was the only female working at night in a room with the ten men responsible for getting the paper out: the typesetters, the press operators and Mr. Sloan. This setup seemed creepy at first, especially when the typesetters snarled at me when I found spelling mistakes. A mistake meant they had to remove that line of type and insert a corrected one. I think most of them wished I didn't know how to spell or use a dictionary. Eventually, we all got along and the men accepted me as part of the team.

Mr. Sloan was the eccentric male counterpart of his wife. I watched him as I sat in my cubicle proofreading. He was probably in his mid-to-late fifties but looked eighty. In charge of the paper's final layout, he stood hunched over a large drafting table with pencil and ruler in hand. He smoked constantly, appeared ashen and sickly and never tapped the ashes off the end of his cigarettes. I watched to see how long the ashes would get before they fell onto his paper layout. If the ashes did fall onto the paper, he just brushed them off and lit another cigarette. When I heard sirens at night, I wondered if the newspaper building had caught fire.

The final layout for the paper was done in the evening to assure that any last minute Associated Press news would make it into the paper. The paper then went to press around midnight. The copies were folded, stacked and ready for delivery by 5:00 the next morning. It was an arduous but amazing process. I was tired, but never bored. In mid-summer, I decreased my Saturday and evening hours to spend more time with Dave.

Our dates that summer revolved around cars. Dave belonged to two sports car clubs in Sacramento which held events on weekends. There were car rallies, races, picnics, shows and swap meets. I found most of these events boring. For hours, the members talked about their cars and drank beer. There was usually a rally scheduled every Sunday during the summer. We alternated cars for these rallies: one week we'd take the XKE, the next, the Corvette. The members met in a prescribed location and rode single-file on a carefully selected, beautiful, winding highway, ending up together at some restaurant where we drank and dined. By the end of summer, I was tired of the car club adventures and glad to return to school.

When a new semester started in the fall, Dave moved back to Sacramento to continue at Sacramento State, and I moved back to Davis for my senior year. I continued working part-time at the Davis paper. When time allowed, I drove home to be of support to my mother. Besta was still in the geriatric ward of the hospital, but her condition was declining. I could hardly stand to see her now. The bright, personable grandmother I had known was morphing into nothingness. If I felt this way, I couldn't imagine how my mother felt.

Dave and I were still dating on weekends, which offset the sadness I felt after seeing my mother and Besta. We no longer participated in the car club activities. With less time devoted to car rallies, we could spend more intimate time together. When the weather was nice, Dave would pack a picnic lunch and we'd drive to some isolated spot in the local hills to enjoy a romantic, peaceful afternoon. On occasional Sundays, we'd put the top down on the car and drive alongside the ocean on Highway 1. Throughout our dating life, Dave remained the kind, considerate gentleman I had dined with at Frank Fat's.

I graduated with a B.A. in English. Though UC Davis had a renowned art program in the 1960s, my father insisted I study a subject that would make me more employable. With my English degree, I dreamed of having a glamorous career as a magazine or book editor, but along with the glamorous dream came the dark nightmare of fear: the deep insecurity spawned by leaving college and the fear of leaving my mother behind. Instead of dwelling on distant dreams, though, I chose to think about the present excitement: Dave had proposed, and we were discussing marriage.

In the fall of 1964, my mother moved Besta into a rest home. My mother was grief-stricken. There was nothing I could do to make her feel better except be there. On many days, Besta neither spoke nor recognized us. It was painful to listen to my mother explain over and over that she was her daughter. "Mom, it's me, your daughter. This is Diane, your granddaughter. We came to see you today. I live here in town. I come every day to make sure that you're treated well here." No response! "Well, I will be going now but will be back tomorrow. I love you mom." These visits were torturous for my mother. Besides wishing she could have a drink, she'd sometimes say, "As bad as it sounds, I wish mom would just die. She has no quality of life and she's suffered enough. Though I hang onto my faith, sometimes I wonder if there really is a loving God out there."

I worked at the newspaper through the summer of 1965. In the fall, I got up the nerve to apply for a job teaching English at a Catholic high school in Sacramento. I got the job at the high school, which happened to be located two blocks from Dave's Sacramento apartment. He was still attending Sacramento State, but never received a degree. He was planning to work on his parents' farm after our wedding.

Dave and I married in February of 1966. The wedding was an extravaganza. The Catholic church was packed and the music was concert quality. My aunt played the harp, my high school Spanish teacher played the organ and a full choir of my high school students sang beautifully in four-part harmony. My father hosted 300 people at the reception which included a sit-down dinner and dancing to a live band. The best gift I received that day was my mother's sobriety. While everyone was toasting and knocking down the drinks, my mother refused to touch a drop of alcohol.

A few days before the wedding, my mother and I went to see Besta. She was lying in bed curled up in the fetal position and completely unresponsive. There was fluid dripping into her vein from an IV bag. When I brushed back her beautiful thick silver hair to kiss her goodbye, I knew I would never see her again. My mother and I walked away crying and I felt sad knowing I would be leaving my mother to go far away on my wedding trip.

Dave and I honeymooned in New York and the Bahamas. We were away for two weeks of fun and relaxation. On our return, Dave's parents met us at the San Francisco airport. We arrived about 4:00p.m. and as we made our way to the luggage carousel, Dave's mother pulled me aside. "I want to tell you that your grandmother died while you were gone. She passed away a few days ago and the rosary is being recited tonight at 7:30. Her funeral is tomorrow morning."

I said, "Why didn't someone call me? I would have come home to be with my mother. I need to leave the airport now so I'll be there for the rosary."

She said, "Nobody called because knowing about her death would have ruined your honeymoon. We can't leave the airport now because I've planned a big dinner party to welcome you and Dave!" She looked at me excitedly. "The airport has a large, glassed in special dining room that I've reserved. I've invited our friends and relatives from the Bay Area and they'll be arriving soon."

Sad and furious, I confronted my mother-in-law. "I don't care about any dinner party. I want to go home to be with my mother."

When I sat down at the table, I told Dave, "I want to go home. Besta's rosary is tonight and if we leave now, we'll be there in time. It's important that I be with my mother."

He responded, "My mother has planned this big party and if we leave, I know how upset she'll be. Besides, we don't have a car. If we take my parents' car, they'll have no way to get home."

I replied, "We could take a taxi and leave your parents here to entertain their guests. After all, it's their party." But Dave wouldn't stand up to his mother and take me home. I was afraid to take a taxi by myself. While the group was drinking and eating, I was seething. My mother paged me three times over the airport intercom while we were partying, begging me to come home. Each time she called she was sobbing, "I need you here. Besta's rosary is tonight. If you leave now you can make it in time." I told her about the dinner and my lack of transportation. Regardless, she kept calling me during dinner, hoping we were on our way. I had no idea if Dave's parents had said anything to her about the dinner party.

The following morning, Dave and I attended Besta's funeral and burial. After the service, my uncle from Alaska told my mother, "Mom had such a hard life and a hard death. After she left dad, she worked so hard to keep us all going. I'll miss her so much. I don't know how I'll live without her." Not long after Besta's death, he died in his early fifties from a stroke. Though the death of her older brother was another loss for my mother, she didn't resort to alcohol to numb the pain. I'm proud of her for that.

PART TWO
Marriage

1966

When I married in February 1966, I was filled with both joy and terror. The Vietnam war was escalating, and Dave, age twenty-five, was prime draft material. It seemed every young man with four functional limbs was being drafted at lightning speed. A week before the wedding, our best man received orders to ship out. I had friends who left the country, got married or went back to school to avoid the draft. Constant reminders of the slaughter reinforced the need to escape. Every newscast showed pictures of wounded men lying in muddy trenches and stacks of flag-draped coffins being loaded onto transport planes.

As I watched pictures of the carnage along with the arrogant and insensitive politicians trying to justify this war, my outrage grew as big and boundless as the war itself. I became obsessed with draft notices, looking through our mail with trepidation for the lethal words "Selective Service." I was terrified. I could barely get food down; my dreams were filled with gruesome war scenes. Dave attempted to ease my fear by trying to convince me that he was not draft material. Without his glasses or contacts, his vision was a blur. Certainly, he reasoned, the military would not send half-blind people into combat! I argued that on the contrary, I had seen pictures of soldiers in battle wearing glasses. His poor vision would keep him from piloting aircraft, but not from crawling in muddy trenches with a machine gun.

At that time I was teaching high school English in Sacramento, a twelve-mile drive from our home in Woodland, California. Dave was driving thirty miles in the opposite direction to work on his family's ranch. We were trying to get pregnant and in late March, when vomiting became part of my morning routine, I discovered I was pregnant. Sick and exhausted, I drove daily to school like a maniac, often nearly late, hoping to make the first bell. This was my pattern until the last Saturday in May when I miscarried. When the cramping started, Dave was in the middle of a field somewhere unreachable. My mother took me to the hospital in Woodland just in time for the fetus to eject under medical supervision. While the doctor cleaned me up, he blabbed on about how common it is for women to miscarry a first pregnancy in the first trimester. He mentioned that some transient residual bleeding might occur which would resolve over time. He made as light of the whole affair as if it were a bowel movement. No mention was made of a D&C procedure, which is frequently done to rid the uterus of any lingering placental tissue which can cause further cramping and bleeding. When finished, he pointed to a small, stainless steel basin and asked casually, "Would you like to know the sex of the fetus?" Jolted by the question, I looked forlornly at the basin and answered,

"Yes." The doctor answered, "It's a boy." It was then that I started to cry. I was struck with the realization that both life and death had occurred within my body. While I was trying to absorb this phenomenon, the doctor interrupted my thoughts with, "You're all set. You can return to work on Tuesday."

Believing in the infallibility of doctors, I went to work on Tuesday. By Thursday, I was still bleeding heavily and could barely drag myself out of bed. I called the doctor who casually stressed the normalcy of the bleeding, reassuring me that it was safe to work. On Friday, I was leaving the classroom every half hour to change my Kotex. By the end of the school day, I looked like a ghost. I was dizzy and felt a heavy weight pulling inside me. With the kind of "help" and "advice" my doctor had been offering, I was reluctant to call him. I had every intention of driving myself home and calling him later, but my colleagues insisted that I call. When I talked to him, he instructed me to "get an ambulance," using the same casual inflection one might use to tell a friend to "get a cab." The ambulance delivered me to our local hospital where the doctor awaited. I had hoped that Dave would be there, but he was working at the ranch and not easily accessible. By the time he did arrive, I was being swiftly discharged with a supply of iron pills. I had lost enough blood to warrant a transfusion, but the doctor assured me that some bed rest and iron would restore me. There was no discussion about a D&C procedure.

With bed rest being the prescription for recovery, I quit teaching. Dave took a week off from work. He shopped, cooked and consoled me. "Don't be upset about losing the baby. Things happen for a reason. Maybe there was something wrong with the fetus and nature, by discharging it, saved the baby from a life of suffering. When you recover, we can try to get pregnant again."

When Dave went back to work, I was still bleeding. I curtailed my physical activity and gave up tennis and swimming. But no matter how much I rested, the bleeding continued. In the mornings when I showered, the blood flowed like a scene from "Psycho." Since the amount of bleeding was directly related to my level of physical activity, I became inactive, cautious and ultimately depressed. While Dave worked at the ranch from sunrise to dusk, I sat home bewildered and frustrated, focusing what energy I had on the mail delivery. I continued to obsess on the mail, rifling frantically through it looking for communication from the draft board. Every day that passed without an envelope from the Selective Service was another day of freedom and relief. Given the inefficiency of government bureaucracy, I hoped that Dave would find obscurity in some overlooked pile of paper.

I spent the summer languishing around the house. Most of my friends had either moved on or were working. Feeling lonely and isolated, I shifted my focus from Vietnam and the draft to Dave's work schedule. Concerned, he had been calling me daily during lunch to check on me and inform me of his location and estimated quitting time. The farm property, which produced almonds, tomatoes and wheat, was spread over many non-adjacent acres. Since I was familiar with the layout, I could picture the fields in relation to his parents' house. Most days, he ate lunch at their home so I knew I could always call to leave him a message or check on his whereabouts. There were no cell phones then, but the field trucks had radios and his mother could always find him. The longer I stayed home alone, the more dependent I became on his phone calls. On days when he didn't call or I couldn't reach his mother, I felt a rush of panic. Trying not to think the worst, I calmed myself with reasonable explanations for their silence: his mother was at the store or Dave couldn't get away for lunch.

One day while feeling more depressed and isolated than usual, I called the ranch with a great need to talk to Dave. His mother, Agnes, answered and informed me that he wasn't around. "Dave drove to Gilroy to pick up a tractor part. Gilroy is about three hours away and Dave has to tow a large piece of equipment back to the ranch. You shouldn't expect him until late evening." When I hung up, I laid on the bed and sobbed. I was consumed by a feeling of abandonment so powerful that I felt like the last person on earth. I called his mother back and asked her to get the name and phone number of the place in Gilroy. Suddenly, my survival seemed to hinge on my ability to contact Dave.

What in the world was wrong with me? I'd never acted this way before. Yes, I felt down about my physical situation, but this was...crazy. His errand was just part of his job, not a catastrophic event. I called the shop in Gilroy and reached Dave, who was sitting around waiting for the part. Hearing the panic in my voice, he called me constantly with updates. He was kind and considerate. On his way home, he stopped regularly at pay phones to give me his location and distance from home. I was frozen to the phone receiver until I knew he was close. When he walked through the door, my fear subsided immediately. Neither of us understood what had triggered my irrational response to his absence. The following day, Dave went back to work and I stayed home with a vague feeling of unease.

In mid-August, I was still bleeding heavily and Agnes, a retired nurse, sprang into action. We were having drinks at the ranch when the subject of my constant bleeding arose. Fueled by a few bourbons and a large financial donation to the hospital, she called the doctor and attacked him mercilessly. "What is wrong with you? This girl has been bleeding for months and you've done nothing about it. The problem could have been solved early on with a D&C. I'm bringing her to the hospital now and you are performing a D&C." Unlike the doctor, she recognized the problem and started the process to solve it. A week after the D&C, the bleeding stopped.

With the doctor's approval, Dave and I attempted another pregnancy. This pregnancy was successful, resulting in the birth of our son, Robert, in June 1967. By the time the baby arrived, I was depleted. Instead of feeling joyful, I was overwhelmed and depressed. I needed rest and time to absorb the impact of motherhood, a role for which I suddenly felt ill-equipped. My state of exhaustion prompted Dave to plan a getaway to Santa Barbara, a place we both loved. In early August, we left the baby with Dave's mother and drove six hours south.

Panic

The road to Solvang is winding and isolated, creeping endlessly through a rugged mountain pass. Solvang, a charming replication of a Danish town, is nestled in the hills about two hours from Santa Barbara. Twenty minutes after leaving Santa Barbara for a day-trip to Solvang, I felt dizzy and nauseous. The more I tried to dismiss these sensations as a natural response to the hairpin twists in the road, the worse I felt. A numbness crept up my arms which riveted my attention on my body. Thinking I was having a heart attack or stroke, I asked Dave to turn around and find a hospital. My breathing felt constricted and the numbness spread throughout my body. Barely able to move my limbs, I was convinced I was dying. By the time we reached a hospital, I was on the verge of passing out. In the emergency room, I was lightly sedated and the numbness abated, allowing me to describe the event to the doctor.

The doctor, a tall, well-dressed Hispanic gentleman, was astute, gentle, and empathetic, his diagnosis casual and simple: "You just hyperventilated. It's a physiological response to a fear-producing situation. The physical sensations you experienced in the car frightened you, causing you to panic and hyperventilate. Hyperventilation is not life-threatening. The worst that can happen when you hyperventilate is that you eventually pass out, but when that happens, your breathing corrects itself and you wake up as though nothing happened."

The doctor's next observations were disturbing. "People hyperventilate for many different reasons. For most, it's just an isolated moment of fear or anxiety that causes the response, but for others, it's the manifestation of deeper emotional problems or the result of either a single traumatic event or a series of them."

Caught completely off-guard by the doctor's insightful comments, I started sobbing. Then I told him about the draft, the miscarriage and the endless bleeding. I was mystified by the quantity of tears, which seemed disproportionate to the events I had been describing. The tears seemed to be a manifestation of something deep, unrecognizable and powerful that dwelled inside, stirred from slumber by the doctor's observation. Years later, after much therapy, I would discover the origin of those tears; but that day in Santa Barbara, they were a mystery.

The doctor discharged me with some Valium to be taken as needed and said, "You have two choices. You can stay and enjoy your vacation or you can go home. There is nothing physically wrong with you. You just reacted to exhaustion, fear and an overload of stress." I left with the Valium but with no real grasp of the connection between fear and hyperventilation and what, if anything, could prevent them.

I had every intention of finishing the vacation, but during the night, I started obsessing about the long ride home, wondering how I was going to make it. I tried to dismiss this thought by telling myself I'd be fine. The drive was days away and I had the Valium to help me. My mind was bombarded by conflicting thoughts, carrying on their own dialogue. *"You love Santa Barbara, you're already here, stay and enjoy your vacation. No, you can't enjoy the vacation because you're dreading the six-hour trip home. After what happened on the Solvang trip, you'll never make six hours. The sooner you leave, the sooner you'll be home and the dreaded car ride will be over."* I was reluctant to tell Dave about my obsessive thoughts. When I tried unsuccessfully to change the subject in my head, I then started obsessing on my inability to control my thoughts. Realizing that I was no longer in control and had lost perspective, I told Dave about my dilemma. He responded with the words I wanted to hear. "There's no sense in staying here and being miserable. Let's pack up and leave. You can take enough Valium to fall asleep in the back seat and I'll drive." Once the decision was made, I couldn't pack fast enough. I needed to leave town immediately. Dave threw our suitcases in the trunk, I took ten milligrams of Valium and we were off.

I slept in the back seat, waking every few hours to check our progress. What had once been innocuous road signs signaling upcoming towns, now became menacing yardsticks for measuring the time and distance from home. Like a kid on a road-trip, I kept asking Dave, "How much longer before we're home?" He would say, "I'm driving as fast as I can. Just relax. We'll be home soon." The closer I got to home, the safer and more relaxed I felt. When we drove into our driveway, I was elated, thoroughly convinced that I had just experienced a very disturbing but "isolated" event. Dave had been tremendously understanding through all this, but I'm sure he hoped the same.

Manipulation

When we returned, the tomato harvest was at its peak and Dave was in the fields from 7:00 a.m. to 8:00 p.m. Since the incident in Santa Barbara, I was afraid to stay home alone for long periods, fearing I'd hyperventilate and there'd be nobody to help me. To avoid the fear, I insisted on going to the ranch with Dave. While he worked, the baby and I stayed with his mother. But after two days in her presence, I knew I had to escape with Dave to the fields. I had never felt comfortable with her and this incarceration proved to me that we had nothing in common and nothing to talk about. She spent her days bragging about her wealth, chain-smoking and reading trashy novels.

But beyond that, there was something elusively strange about her. Even her husband, Don, seemed to avoid her by spending every day at the golf course playing the same nine holes over and over. He came home just in time to have a few strong bourbons, eat and go to bed.

Dave was an only child who had been brought up by these people who made no sense to me. In turn, I made no sense to them when I chose to sit in Dave's hot pickup all day while he drove a tractor. Finding the boredom worse than the heat, I learned to drive a tractor. Dave and I finished tomato harvest together, returning each evening to the ranch for dinner.

By the end of the harvest, Dave was frustrated with his role in the family's farming operation. He was tired of driving a tractor and being assigned mundane tasks by Hank, the tenant who had farmed the property for years. While Hank received a large share of the crop proceeds, Dave punched a time clock and Hank paid him the same hourly wage as the other laborers. Dave had asked Hank for more responsibility, but he ignored Dave's request. Dave then went to his parents. Over dinner one evening with his parents, Dave raised the issue. "I'm tired of working for Hank as a laborer. I'd like to have more control over the farm operation, especially the choice of crops that are planted. Hank just plants the same crops over and over. I've learned by watching other farmers that there are more lucrative crops that would do well here. Hank's afraid to try anything new. I asked Hank for more responsibility, but he ignored me. Now, I'm asking you and mom, the landowners, to help me out by discussing the matter with Hank." Dave's parents reluctantly agreed to talk to Hank.

A week later, the verdict was in. Over drinks, Don said to Dave, "Your mother and I have talked to Hank and we have to go along with his thinking. Hank is worried that your lack of experience would jeopardize crop production and income. Hank has been farming our land for years and we've always made a good living off the crop proceeds. We don't want to risk losing Hank or our income. Remember, Hank was farming the property when your great-aunt owned it, long before your mother inherited the land. Now, let's eat!"

Dave was hurt, angry and discouraged by his parents' lack of trust and support. With innovative ideas and an innate enjoyment of farming, Dave would have been a good farmer. But with no opportunity to pursue new methods and ideas and no increase in pay, Dave quit. Feeling betrayed by his parents, he walked away defeated and depressed.

Though Dave missed farming, we were happy to be home together. Now that he was home every day, I could be free of the constant anxiety of wondering what field he was in and whether I could reach him. His presence also gave me a respite from dwelling on my fear of being home alone for long periods of time. The only time I was alone now was when Dave ran local errands and I stayed home with the baby. Since we lived in the small town where I grew up, I knew the location of the stores in relation to our house; this knowledge gave me a sense of comfort and security. It was a happy and peaceful time, the kind of time that naive youth believes will last forever.

A year into this idyllic scene, the issue of money dragged us into reality. The longer Dave stayed home, the more curious I became about our finances. I presumed he had a plan for bringing in money, but when nothing evolved, I was baffled. He assured me there was no need to worry about money because he received a percentage of the farm income. His explanation was vague, and I noticed no checks ever arrived in the mail. When our bank balance dwindled, he called his mother and large sums of money miraculously appeared in our account. There seemed to be no limit to requests or resources and his mother never questioned how the money was spent. Dave bought me expensive clothes and jewelry while his closet was full of hand-tailored suits, silk ties and Italian shoes. We drove expensive cars. His mother had written the check for our "executive" style home and paid the local "decorator" to furnish it. Though I never questioned the existing financial arrangement, I thought it peculiar. I remained silent because I believed that Dave's arrangement with his mother was none of my business. Besides, I didn't want to appear mistrustful of Dave.

Whenever the subject of looking for work came up in front of Dave's mother, her response was always, "You kids don't need to worry about money; there is plenty of money from the ranch and you'll always be taken care of." To her, work was not a wholesome, gratifying endeavor. It was a negative four-letter word which only applied to the unfortunates who hadn't inherited money. She couldn't fathom the idea that anyone who already had money might actually want to work. She was unlike anyone I had ever met. Everyone I knew worked, including wealthy people. Her attitudes exacerbated my discomfort, and led me to question her motives. I didn't believe she showered us with money out of love and generosity. Instead, I saw her as a dominant, controlling woman who used her money and distorted work philosophy to control her husband, her son and now me. Her unspoken message was, "Don't worry about working and becoming independent of me, just let

me be boss in exchange for a lifetime of financial security."
My innate suspicion of her added to the ever-widening
emotional gap between us.

In spite of his mother, Dave and I continued to discuss
his need to find some kind of work. I believed the success
of our marriage hinged on our financial independence, but
every time we discussed the matter, Dave got uncomfortable.
He'd never worked anywhere but on the family farm. He
was reluctant to take charge of the situation, and seemed
lost and scared.

To counter Dave's mother's power of dissuasion, my
father, whose vocation was selling life insurance, had an
avocation of managing other peoples' lives. He called on
a regular basis to check on Dave's job status. He usually
called between seven and eight in the morning with the
same message, "What in the hell are you doing in bed? You
should be out looking for a job. If you can't find a job, I'll
find one for you." While Dave's mother couldn't fathom
why anyone with money would want to work, my father
couldn't understand anyone *not* wanting to work. He loved
work for its own sake and believed that his relentless attacks
would motivate Dave.

Growing weary of my father's calls and unsolicited
advice, Dave decided to buy a fast-food franchise. While
his parents were willing and ready to write the check for
the purchase, my father intervened upon hearing about
the idea. Based on Dave's lack of business experience and
motivation, he convinced Dave's parents that purchasing
a food franchise was financial idiocy. Instead, my father

offered what he considered the perfect solution to Dave's job dilemma: One of his friends was selling his florist shop and would be willing to teach Dave the business. With no input from Dave or me, his parents, abetted by my father, purchased the florist shop. Dave and I should have headed for the hills, leaving the folks to run the business, but we had unwittingly become compliant pawns in the hands of master manipulators. Perhaps they were well-meaning manipulators, but manipulators nevertheless.

Escalating Fear

Dave started his apprenticeship at the business while I stayed home with the baby. I was still uncomfortable being home without Dave but I quelled my fear by thinking of ways to manage it or escape from it. I told myself that the flower shop was only minutes away and Dave could be home quickly if I needed him. If I started to feel anxious or focus obsessively on my breathing and hyperventilation, I could distract myself with chores. If I became overwhelmed by fear and Dave couldn't leave the shop, I could drive there. It took tremendous effort and focus to keep the fear submerged.

The longer I stayed home alone beating down my fear, the more constant and intrusive the feeling of panic and fear of hyperventilation became. The calming effect of phoning Dave or doing chores wore off more quickly. As time passed, I feared more situations. The minute I stepped into a grocery store, I could hardly wait to get out. I dashed around the store in a state of panic hurriedly snatching the immediate necessities from the shelves. I found the shortest checkout line and told the clerk I wasn't feeling well and needed to get out of the store quickly. Going to the grocery store by myself became so traumatic that Dave took over the shopping. I could go with him, but I couldn't go alone.

The same fear of standing in line and worrying about hyperventilating happened at the bank, the movies and concerts. I felt trapped standing in line at the bank and stuck while in the middle of a transaction. I could still go to concerts and movies but I could no longer sit in the middle of a row of seats: I had to sit next to the aisle to assure a quick escape. Getting the right seat at the show meant arriving at least forty minutes ahead so I could be first in line. My escalating fear took on a domino effect: Previously safe places kept toppling one after the other. I began avoiding crowds and busy stores fearing that I would lose sight of Dave in the crowd. I avoided large buildings where I might become disoriented or an easy escape might be compromised. Almost every activity now required careful scrutiny as the criteria imposed by my anxiety and fear of hyperventilation began to shrink my world. The need to meet such strict criteria made me feel stressed, defeated and helpless. I worried about whether our son could sense and absorb my high level of stress.

Though I was still able to drive around town by myself, the thought of driving alone on the freeway became terrifying and inconceivable. I could drive or ride anywhere with Dave because I felt safe with him; he understood how frightened I was, and his presence ensured the availability of help. He was my rock. I had family and friends in town, but was too ashamed to confide in them. Besides, I had no way to define the situation; it was nameless.

As my fear and avoidance worsened, my self-esteem diminished and my depression increased. I became more anxious and controlling. I had no idea what was happening to me; I blamed myself for my increasing fear. My first scare had come in Santa Barbara while riding in a car. At that time, I considered the incident to be an isolated event, not something that would expand into a life-altering monster. In addition to the blame and shame I was now heaping on myself, I began lamenting and dwelling on the things I had previously done with ease, wondering where my competent self had gone.

The person I used to be had driven all over California, ridden the train and made numerous trips by air. Dave and I honeymooned in New York and the Bahamas. Every step onto a plane or into a car had been filled with excitement, not fear. I wanted my old self back. I didn't like or know the person I had become. I needed help and information. I searched the library for clues about my symptoms but found nothing. There would be nothing helpful until I entered into therapy several years later. In the meantime, I tried to appear "normal" by focusing on the baby, Dave and the flower shop.

1970

One morning I received an unprecedented call from the manager of our flower shop. There was panic and urgency in his voice. "Diane, you must come down to the store immediately. There's something I need to show you." I asked for specifics but he said, "You must come see for yourself." When I arrived, Dave was in the office with the door shut. The manager led me to a set of large drawers behind the sales counter. He opened them and I looked quizzically inside. "Unpaid bills," he told me. "Every one of them. This business is going down the tubes." I saw stacks and stacks of unopened envelopes. Most of them were from wholesalers and government agencies. Months of payroll and sales taxes were overdue and the unpaid balances were accumulating large amounts of penalties and interest. There was a notice from the State Board of Equalization threatening to close the store. I was speechless. I didn't need a degree in accounting to know this was a dire situation.

I tapped on the office door. Dave opened it, surprised, and joined the manager and me behind the counter.

"Dave," I said as gently as I could, "these bills. How did—how did this...?"

Dave's expression changed from surprise to terror to shame.

I felt my own fear rise. "Why didn't you tell me?"

He hung his head and stared for a long time at the floor. I could tell he was fighting back tears. He finally said, "We're just not making enough money. I can't pay any of them. I thought I could fix it before you found out." He bit his lip. "Meanwhile, I just shoved everything out of sight."

The problem now was owning the mess and finding a solution. We set up a nursery in the office and I went to the store daily. Dave and I opened every envelope together, separating the contents by date, type and urgency. In addition to the accumulated unpaid sales tax, the State Board of Equalization was requiring us to fund a reserve account determined by a percentage of our delinquent amount. This reserve would be used by the board to fund future late payments. If we stayed current for a pre-determined amount of years, the board would release the money. The sum of all the debt totaled about sixty-thousand dollars, an astonishing amount for 1970 and twenty-thousand more than we had paid for the business.

Our options were to walk away in disgrace or beg Dave's parents for the money. Not knowing what else to do, we chose the latter. His parents wrote out a check for the entire debt plus additional money for working capital. Dave's father was furious and a running commentary about responsibility ensued. My father jumped into the fray, blaming Dave's parents for raising a spoiled, lazy child who had no regard for money. I felt bad for Dave because he seemed lost and dazed. He was passive and sad, like a kid being bullied on the playground. Wanting to help, I learned bookkeeping and took over the job. For different reasons, Dave and I were happy working together. He appreciated my help and I was no longer stuck home with only three-year-old Robert for company.

As bookkeeper, I discovered Dave was right about the shortfall of revenue. All along, I had presumed the store was providing us with a living, but all the money was going to overhead and over-buying. After learning of the revenue shortage, I wondered how Dave was making ends meet at home. Since we still had a working phone and electricity, I presumed everything was fine. I was dismayed to learn that Dave's parents still remained the source of our income, even for our personal life.

Then one morning I was awakened at six a.m. by a deafening banging and clanking outside. I ran to the window in time to see our year-old Buick Riviera being towed down the street by a repo company. Dave dismissed the repo as "no big deal"—he'd just forgotten to make the payments. His parents put up the money to bail the car out, and Dave promised to be more financially vigilant.

I didn't understand the way we were living. Friends our age had professions or jobs and were self-reliant. We were a kept couple and I resented Dave's parents, their strange relationship with their son, and their willingness to foster his dependence. Though the interaction between Dave and his parents was unfathomable to me, I did understand that to be free, we had to become autonomous. But the thought of autonomy frightened both of us. Dave was too insecure to risk independence and my fear of panic kept me tied to familiar surroundings. Our separate fears left us stuck and vulnerable to the control and needs of our intrusive parents, driving me deeper into the feelings of panic and helplessness I was trying to ignore.

My Mother's Keeper

By early 1971, my anxiety, panic and avoidance had escalated to the point where Dave and I were inseparable. We were like two flimsy playing cards leaning on each other for support. He was my panic support person and I was his business support. We worked together, played tennis together, and ran every errand together, hauling Robert and his diaper bag along. Family and friends joked about our togetherness. We had no individual freedom and nothing new to bring to the relationship. We survived by ignoring the problems, and pretending we were in charge of our lives.

In March, I became pregnant with our second son. On the mornings I was sick, Dave stayed home with me. On those occasions, my father would call to tell us how lazy we were. When Dave told him I was pregnant and sick, his response was, "Go to work without her. You don't need to hold her hand. You need to get your ass out of bed and go to work." If I had been foolish enough to explain my daily state of panic to my father, he would have released a barrage of ridicule, driving me further into secrecy and hiding.

Moreover, my problems were irrelevant to my parents. They needed me to be available to listen to their marital problems, expecting me to take sides or fix them. The situation was never reversed. I kept my pain and problems to myself.

My parents' behavior stretched beyond the limits of self-involvement. It was erratic and scary. I had been a captive of their dysfunction for most of my life. For example, when I was fifteen, my father began leaving our home in Woodland for days at a time. He never told us where he was going, when he would return or how to reach him. He always left my mother with sufficient money to sustain us. His method of departure was always the same: He would wait until no one was home, take some clothes, and leave a lengthy letter on the piano addressed to my mother and us three children. In the letter he would rant about his unhappy marriage, my mother's problems, and his need to get away to "sort things out."

My mother expected me, as the oldest of the three kids to look after her and my siblings. During these absences, my mother drank heavily, which was a practice that rendered her useless and fueled her depression. While she sobbed in her room, I would spend hours with her trying to talk her out of her misery and back into being functional. Propping my mother up during these episodes was a full-time job and one that stretched the emotional limits of a teenager. When I became frustrated and frightened by her depression and inertia, I sought solace by spending evenings and weekends with my paternal grandmother and my aunt. But there was no end to this crazy, erratic behavior. It continued throughout my parents' lives.

One of the more frightening examples of this behavior occurred in the summer of 1971. Though my mother had quit drinking in 1961, she remained emotionally vulnerable to my father's controlling and belittling behavior. Terrified to be home alone, she had relied on the presence of her children. But in 1971, when my father left again, none of us children were living at home. My mother, who for years had been stashing a portion of her grocery stipend, hired a private detective to track down my father. When she discovered that he was living with a woman in a nearby town, she came undone, spiraling into a deep, dark depression. Feeling responsible and sad for her, for the next several months I checked on her daily and brought her over for dinner. When she was with me and Dave, she ate very little and talked about suicide. Just before bedtime, Dave, I and our toddler took her home and turned on her lights. She insisted that Dave check all the closets, under the beds and in the basement to make sure no one was hiding. On the nights when she refused to come over or answer the phone, Dave, I and our son went to her house. If nobody answered the door, I dreaded going inside, picturing her lying lifeless on the floor from an overdose or a gunshot wound. When we got up the nerve to go inside, we would creep fearfully from room to room, turning on lights, praying we wouldn't find her body.

By early summer, my mother looked dreadful. She refused to eat and kept talking about wishing she were dead. Feeling compelled to get help and unable to locate my father, Dave and I took her to the hospital where she was admitted to the psychiatric ward. She remained there medicated for three weeks either asleep or sitting dazed in the day room. Visiting consisted of sitting and staring with her and the other blank patients. To keep from panicking, I kept telling myself that unlike the patients, I was free to leave any time. Seeing my mother sitting unresponsively in a stupor depressed and frightened me. I hated to leave her and I hated to return for visits. Recognizing the similarity between her fears and mine, I wondered if genetics would lead me to a similar fate.

My father was back home when my mother was released from the hospital. She was prescribed an antidepressant and weekly follow-up appointments with a psychiatrist. She disliked the doctor but continued to see him to get prescription refills. By October, she had quit seeing the doctor and taking her pills. Because I had never seen much improvement in her depression, I wondered if she had ever taken the pills and whether the doctor was paying attention.

In late October of 1971, my father left home again. When he returned late one evening to get something he needed, he found my mother lying on the living room couch. Noticing that she was in an uncomfortable position, he tried to wake her. When she failed to respond to repeated proddings, he called an ambulance. At 11:30, he called to tell me that she was unconscious in ICU. Dave and I raced to the hospital to find my father and sister sitting in the waiting room. No visitors were allowed in ICU in those days, so we sat and waited for the doctor to appear with his prediction of a bad outcome. While my sister and I cried, my father fell asleep.

To increase our mother's chance of survival, the doctor wanted to know what drug she had taken. He insisted that one of us go to the house and look through the garbage for an empty prescription bottle. Since I was eight months pregnant and my father was asleep, my sister went at 12:30 to rummage through the garbage. She returned with an empty container labeled Tofranil, her antidepressant medication. Who knows how much she had taken? At 2:00 a.m., the doctor told us to go home, promising to keep us informed. Miraculously, my mother woke up at 8:00 the following morning. Because organ damage was a possible side effect of the overdose, she spent a week under observation in the regular section of the hospital. After being declared physically healthy, she was moved to the psychiatric ward for another two weeks.

By the time my second son, Stephen, was born in November, our lives had returned to the previous normal. My father was home and my mother was doing her best to maintain her equilibrium. Her spirits had been lifted by her sister-in-law, who encouraged her to stand up for herself by threatening divorce. Though my mother would never have gone through with a divorce, just the mention of the "D" word subdued my father considerably. The last thing he wanted was a publicly tarnished image, the loss of half his assets, spousal support and the loss of control.

During this time of family stress, Dave and I spent little time at the flower shop. Our competent staff managed the still struggling store in our absence. At the start of 1972, Dave and I returned to work full-time. In spite of my unresolved fear and avoidance issues, the potential for some order and consistency in our lives seemed possible. During this period of relative calm, Dave and I bought another flower shop located in Davis, the home of the University of California, Davis. The store, only eight miles from Woodland, was successful; it added more revenue than expense to our struggling original operation. Thankfully, there was a manager in place who was capable of running the store without constant oversight.

But in 1974, two years after the new purchase, Dave became disenchanted with the flower business. To him, the low profits didn't justify the demanding and tedious work. He began to hate the store, staying home from work and questioning his desire and ability to keep the business. Dave, who never complained or blamed, began blaming my father and his parents for dumping the business on us. His anger and indifference resounded in the repeated statement, "For all I care, the business and my parents can go to hell! I wish we'd never bought the store, but we got trapped into it by our know-it-all asshole parents. I wish we could just move out of town and leave the shop and parents behind."

Knowing Dave wanted out of the business gave my father and his parents another opportunity to interfere, criticize and blame. I was tired of the entire situation, growing angrier about my panic attacks and the financial dependency that kept us from escaping. I was losing confidence in Dave's financial and emotional ability to care for me and the kids. This lack of confidence increased my fear and anxiety.

I agreed with Dave about the parent issue. "Your parents and my father, thinking they were doing us a big favor, set us up in the flower shop. Neither of us even had a say about it. How did we let this happen? I wish I didn't have my panic problem and that you had a way to make a living. I'd like to get out of here too, but I don't see it happening. I'm not sure either one of us is emotionally equipped to survive a change."

Just the mention of relocating prompted Dave's mother to say, "If you move away, you'll never get another dime from me." Additionally, since my mother's suicide attempt, I felt responsible for keeping her safe. Foolishly, I believed that my proximity and vigilance would ensure her safety. After eight years of marriage, we were still emotionally and financially trapped by the same players and problems. Unable to run away, the escape that we chose was to sell the original flower shop. We kept the newly purchased store in Davis, but removed ourselves from the daily operation by giving the manager control and an option to buy the business.

PART THREE
Dissolution of Marriage

Ellen

My life changed unexpectedly and dramatically in the summer of 1975, when one of our guests brought a friend with her to dinner. The friend, Ellen, was a nurse who had recently moved from the Midwest to San Francisco, eighty miles from where Dave and our family lived in Woodland. Our mutual friend was leaving town for the summer and hoped that by introducing Ellen to us, Ellen would have new friends to visit while she was gone. Dave and I liked Ellen, who soon became a regular weekend guest. I was attracted to Ellen because she had traits that I admired and envied. She was gregarious, independent, and self-sufficient. She had put herself through nursing school, left her hometown in Ohio and moved wherever and whenever she wanted, never questioning her ability to adapt or make a new life for herself. This type of independence and self-sufficiency was an enigma to me, and I envied her fearlessness and freedom. When I was with her, I felt soothed by the feelings of safety, strength and comfort that she emanated. We liked the same books and music and could spend hours playing duets on the piano or sitting by the pool discussing a book. Between visits, I was sad and lonely. I lived for her next visit, confused and frightened by the longing that I felt.

One evening after Dave, Ellen and I had been out to dinner, I stopped in Ellen's bedroom to chat, while Dave stumbled upstairs to bed. All of us had drunk too much. I was sitting on her bedroom floor freezing in my pajamas and she was lying in bed. When I complained about being cold, Ellen invited me to join her in bed. I accepted the invitation. With the alcohol erasing our inhibitions, the unspoken attraction and longing we had for each other became unleashed. When the morning light appeared, I scurried upstairs and climbed into bed with Dave. As I watched him sleep, I was overcome by the bewilderment and shock resulting from my disloyal and aberrant behavior. I couldn't remember whether Ellen or I initiated the first contact or how it escalated; it just happened.

When the three of us ate breakfast together the next morning, I didn't know what to expect. Frightened and ashamed, I avoided eye contact with Ellen. I wondered if Dave had any inkling of what had transpired between me and Ellen. I wondered how Ellen felt. I needed to know: I had to talk to her. I got my chance when Dave went outside after breakfast. After Dave left, Ellen said, "I was scared to death last night. I didn't know whether Dave knew you weren't in bed and might come looking for you. I was afraid he was going to burst into the room and things would turn ugly. I really care for you but find this situation uncomfortable and frightening." Regardless of what either Ellen or I said, I knew that the relationship between me and Dave and me and Ellen had taken on a new dynamic and that our lives would never be the same.

Though I knew something dramatic had happened between me and Ellen, I had no idea what to call it. One day, a sample copy of a Catholic newspaper came in the mail. The headline on the front page was, "Catholic Church Bans Homosexuality." The article immediately grabbed my attention and as I read it, I was stunned. It included descriptions of homosexual behavior and the words "lesbian" and "gay." The only word I'd ever heard relevant to this subject was "queer." In high school, our masculine-looking girls' P.E. teacher was always referred to as queer. Throughout the hallways, the high school jocks and idiots used the word as the highest form of insult and derision. Now this loathsome word seemed to apply to me. I needed more information, and I needed it quickly.

I went to the dictionary and the encyclopedia but found the most thorough discussion in my paperback copy of Simone de Beauvoir's classic, *The Second Sex*. Every day I surreptitiously read those pages over and over trying to absorb their meaning and to decide if the words really applied to me. I didn't understand how I could be a lesbian and still be attracted to men. Dave and I had always had a good physical relationship, but now I was attracted to Ellen. I was perplexed. I didn't want Ellen to leave and I didn't want to leave Dave or hurt him in any way. How did I get into this mess and what was I going to do? Was I in love with Ellen? With Dave? With both? What was I? I had no idea where we were all headed but I was troubled by the trajectory.

Due to the guilt and fear we both felt after our first night together, Ellen and I abstained from further physical contact. She continued to spend her free time with me and Dave, making for an awkward threesome. During our time apart, Ellen and I missed each other terribly, but we communicated almost daily by phone and mail.

In the summer of 1976, a year after meeting Ellen, she moved to our town. She wanted to buy a home, but knew she couldn't afford anything in San Francisco. She bought a condo in Woodland and got a job at the local hospital. I had been too embarrassed to tell her about my panic problem, so when we visited, I made sure it was always at my house. The added stress of my sexual dilemma exacerbated my fear and anxiety. There was nobody I could talk to. I didn't feel I could tell Ellen about my panicky feelings and I just couldn't tell Dave about my feelings for Ellen. My head was spinning with confusion. What I really wanted to do was go away by myself for a few weeks to a retreat or someplace where I could find help to sort out my life. But my fear of leaving home and my unwillingness to share my feelings left me on my own, groping around in the dark.

Homo, Hetero and Bi

Ellen was the person I wanted Dave to be. The difference between them was glaring and disturbing. The safety and security that I felt with Ellen was different from the financially comfortable life that Dave and I were living. Ellen was a practical person living in the real world with a real job. She was not being bankrolled or controlled by anyone. When Dave quit the flower shop, I presumed he would look for a new line of work. It never happened. It didn't need to happen because his mother kept funneling money into our account. Ellen, by contrast, was in charge of her life and confident of her skills. I wanted Dave to be strong and in charge. I wanted him to be a proud provider and strong enough to get his mother and my father out of our lives. I wanted our family to be separate and self-sufficient, not part of someone else's plan. I loved Dave but I didn't like the way we lived. I didn't know how to make our lives work as individuals or as a couple. The thought of leaving him and disrupting our family terrified me. Divorce was also against my core beliefs of honoring vows and working through problems.

With so much confusion and so much at stake, I knew we needed help. I told Dave that while I still loved him, I was also attracted to Ellen. But Dave refused to discuss Ellen. I had no idea how much he knew about my relationship with her. I chalked up his unwillingness to talk about the matter to his "head-in-the-sand" mentality. But when I explained that our marriage was at risk, Dave reluctantly agreed to see a therapist.

One of Ellen's San Francisco friends suggested we see Dr. Wardell Pomeroy, a clinical psychologist who for twenty years had worked closely with Dr. Alfred Kinsey of the Kinsey Institute. In 1976, Dr. Pomeroy had relocated to San Francisco to become the academic dean of the Institute for Advanced Study of Human Sexuality. When I called for an appointment, he was reluctant to see us because his work with the institute didn't allow much time for individual counseling. But I convinced him that I was struggling with my sexual identity and the future of my marriage. Fortunately, he agreed to see the three of us. I panicked at the thought of driving to San Francisco for therapy, but convinced myself that I would be safe with both Dave and Ellen in the car. Though Ellen knew nothing about my panic problem, I was comfortable with her and trusted her ability to help me if I started to hyperventilate.

We began therapy in the summer of 1976, about a month after Ellen moved to Woodland. Our sessions took place in Dr. Pomeroy's office which was in his home, one of San Francisco's old Victorians. He met us at the door and welcomed us into his living room. The room was full of bookcases overflowing with books and papers. Oriental carpets were scattered over hardwood floors upon which sat big, old furniture with doilies on the arms. The house was eerily quiet, the only sound coming from a ticking clock.

Dr. Pomeroy matched the house. He was quiet, scholarly and direct, and wore the tweed, patched- elbow coat associated with academia. As the three of us sat rigidly on the couch, he pulled up a chair across from us and took a few minutes to silently assess each of us. He then made it clear that he knew why we were there based on my phone request for help. He explained his protocol for therapy. His plan would consist of weekly visits for a time to be determined by his assessment of progress. During our time in therapy, he would see us individually, in pairs and the three of us together. He emphasized that he was primarily a sex therapist and his goal was to give us information that would help us find a direction.

One of the first things he presented to us individually was Dr. Kinsey's Heterosexual-Homosexual Rating Scale. The scale is a method of self-evaluation based on individual experience. The numbers on the scale range from zero through six with zero representing exclusively heterosexual desire and experience and six exclusively homosexual. There are gradations of sexual behavior and desire between the numbers one through five, with the number three representing equally heterosexual and homosexual desire and experience. The purpose of the scale, which was developed by Kinsey and his colleagues in 1948, was to account for their research findings which showed that people didn't fit neatly into exclusively heterosexual or homosexual categories. The research attempted to dispel the myth that sexual

behavior is black or white, right or wrong, normal or abnormal by showing that gradations exist.

In our individual sessions, he explained the rating scale
to each of us and asked us where we thought we fit on the
scale and to describe the feelings and experiences on which
we based our decision. After our individual rating sessions,
he met with us together. He said, "Based on the information
each of you provided, I would rate Ellen a five, Dave a
zero and Diane a three. This means Ellen is predominantly
homosexual, Dave is exclusively heterosexual and Diane is
bisexual. This presents a dilemma for all of you. Dave and
Ellen want to be with Diane, and Diane wants to be with
Dave and Ellen. To help each of you sort out your feelings,
I'm requesting that for three weeks, Diane alternates
between spending four consecutive nights with Dave and
three nights with Ellen. During the intimate time you
share, I want each of you to pay close attention to your
thoughts and feelings. Hopefully, this exercise will help you
determine a direction. I'll see all of you in three weeks to
see how things are going."

The entire situation seemed strange and awkward to
the three of us. Dave became sullen on the nights I was
with Ellen, but never discussed the matter. I had hoped he
would fight for our marriage. A part of me wanted him to
beg me not to leave him. But, his distance and silence left
the burden of making a decision up to me. When finished
with this experiment, the original dilemma still remained.
I thought how much easier it would be if I were strictly
heterosexual or homosexual, not stuck in the middle
attracted to both sexes.

Now I faced two dilemmas: What was I going to do about my marriage and my children? How could I transition into a different way of living while I was still fearful and panicky?

Unfortunately, the subject of my panic didn't come up during therapy. I was afraid to introduce the topic. Dr. Pomeroy had made it clear at the onset that his practice was limited to sexual matters and I didn't want to cross the line. After five weeks, with nothing resolved, our therapy ended. Dr. Pomeroy assured us that in time we would find a direction and emphasized that a resolution would bring peace of mind. He also reassured us that we were not freaks. We were part of the broad spectrum of human sexuality that is misunderstood by people who don't want to believe in gradations of sexual behavior.

Unhinged

When therapy ended, Dave and I tried to return to our previous life but things just weren't the same. Even after therapy, he was still unwilling to discuss our unresolved situation. In the evenings, he began drinking more heavily, which frightened me. Though he was usually even-tempered, from time to time he would fly into a scary, irrational rage after he had been drinking. I was giving up hope that he and I could have a rational discussion about our relationship.

Because I blamed myself for creating our marriage dilemma, I felt a painful compulsion to choose between Dave and Ellen. My ambivalence was keeping everyone in limbo. Unable to ignore or hide my feelings for Ellen, I moved in with her in the late summer of 1976, strictly on a trial basis. I expected Dave to be either furious or sad about my decision but he remained calm and compliant. Since it was understood that I would be living with Ellen on a trial basis, I kept most of my belongings at Dave's house. With a key to the house, advance notice and Dave's encouragement, I went in and out of the house at will. For a while, he and I maintained a cordial relationship.

When my parents learned I had moved in with Ellen, they became unhinged. My "lesbianism" became the subject of our small town gossip and the family embarrassment. My father's entire focus now shifted to destroying my relationship with Ellen. He used a variety of tactics to attempt this.

On a fall morning in 1976, Ellen and I were at Dave's when my father pulled up in his yellow Cadillac. I panicked! I asked Dave to answer the door and tell my father I wasn't there. My father responded, "Don't give me that crap. I know she's here. Tell her I have some important papers for her in the car where I'll be waiting for her. I'm not leaving until I show her what I have." I knew he'd sit there all day or bang nonstop on the front door, so I figured it was better to meet him and get it over with. Afraid that he'd try to kidnap me, I told Dave to watch from the window. I got into the front passenger seat and left the door open. He had a pile of papers on the front seat and explained, "I hired a private detective to do a background check on Ellen. These papers are the detective's report. You might like to read them. According to the report, Ellen is an escapee from a mental institution in Ohio." He held the papers up. "It's all right here. You're making a big mistake hanging around with her."

I couldn't believe this was happening. I said, "You're out of your mind. I'm not interested in your phony report.

This is one of the most asinine things I've ever heard. If this is your idea of help, I don't need it. I want you to leave me alone." I slammed the car door and went back into the house. Dave and Ellen were incredulous when I told them what had happened.

In November of 1976, a month after the private detective incident, Ellen's father died. She went to Ohio for the funeral and I stayed with Dave. While she was gone, my father went to the hospital with the intention of getting Ellen fired. He told the nursing director that he represented Dave's mother, Agnes, who would like to file a complaint against the hospital for hiring Ellen, a lesbian. The nursing director, also a lesbian, told him that if Dave's mother had a complaint, she'd have to present it herself. After he left the hospital, the nurse phoned Dave's mother to inform her of the incident. Furious, Agnes called my father. "The hospital called to tell me you used my name to file a complaint. Don't you ever do that again or I'll take legal action."

When Ellen returned to work, she was informed of my father's attempt to get her fired. Already distraught over her father's death, she now feared for her job. The nursing director, who was smart, respected and understood the fear of being an exposed lesbian, convinced Ellen that her job was safe.

With all of his efforts to destroy Ellen's credibility backfiring, my father resorted to a new level of intimidation. He bragged to me that he could hire a "hit man" for five-thousand dollars to take care of Ellen. In an attempt to fight back, I told him, "If something happens to Ellen, you'd be the first suspect. I'd tell the police what you just told me and you'd end up in prison." After this threat, Ellen watched her back every time she left the hospital.

The next lunatic assault occurred early on a Saturday morning at Ellen's condo. It was Ellen's day off and we were both asleep when someone started beating on the front door. Ellen threw on her clothes and ran downstairs to look through the peephole. There stood my father. I could hear the loud conversation. Ellen said, "What do you want?"

"I want to talk to my daughter."

"Well, she's asleep, but I'll see if she wants to talk to you."

"What do you mean you'll see if she wants to talk to me? I'm her father and she better want to talk to me!"

Ellen ran upstairs. "Your father's at the door demanding to talk to you."

I was so upset I was shaking. "Tell him I don't want to talk to him." Ellen, seeing how upset I was said, "Don't worry. I'll give him the message and get rid of him."

When Ellen relayed my message, my father became furious. "I don't believe she won't talk to me. I don't trust you. I think you're holding her hostage here. If you don't open this door, I'll break it down."

Hearing the commotion, I looked down from the top of the stairs. My father was pushing against one side of the door while Ellen was pushing against the other. He got the door open, but was stopped by the door-chain. Ellen yelled at him, "If you break into this house, I'll call the police.

Now get out of here. No one breaks into my house."

He finally left. Ellen was furious, but I was terrified. Ellen said, "Don't be afraid of him. He's just a bully. I should go to the police and explain what happened. Maybe if they haul him into the station, he'll realize there are consequences for threatening and bullying people."

A few hours later, Ellen did go to the police. They called my father into the station and warned him about trespassing, threatening an arrest if he persisted. After his encounter with the police, he stopped this aggressive form of harassment.

The circus never ended. When my father wasn't performing, my mother and Dave's parents were busy convincing my sons, who were nine and five, that Ellen was a monster who had taken me away from them. They portrayed me as a mindless zombie living under the spell of a master hypnotist. As a result of their propaganda, my children became afraid to stay with me or Ellen. There wasn't a glimmer of support, understanding or compassion. With the exception of an ongoing, somewhat civil relationship with Dave, Ellen and I lived in exile.

Dave hoped that I would eventually return home and didn't want to shut the door in my face. He was also being mercilessly attacked by my father for his inability to stand up for himself. My father berated him for being weak, spineless and too passive to take charge of the situation. "Why are you putting up with Ellen? You need to kick her out of your life. She's ruining your marriage and destroying your family." My father wanted Dave on his side, but Dave was tired of being bullied by him. Ironically, to spite my father, Dave stood up for me and Ellen, creating a mutual alliance against my father.

The Unraveling

When I first moved in with Ellen, she was working the day shift, seven to three-thirty. Somehow, in my state of total confusion, I hadn't thought about how I was going to cope with being alone while she worked. With Dave, I had managed by structuring our lives so we were inseparable. This survival tactic would not work with Ellen's hospital job. Fearful that Ellen would leave me if she knew I was afraid to stay home alone or could only drive a few miles by myself, I needed a strategy that would allow me to look like a normal, independent person.

My first ploy was to tell Ellen I needed the car while she was at work. The pretense was to drop her off, return home and pick her up later. Instead, I dropped her off and stayed parked all day in the hospital lot where I would be close to her. If I got uncomfortable or needed the bathroom, I went into the hospital lobby. I avoided eating in the hospital cafeteria for fear of running into her. For lunch I would either go without or get up the nerve to go to the fast-food restaurant down the street. When Ellen got into the car after work, she presumed that I had just arrived. This behavior went on for several weeks until it became unbearable. I had to move on to a more comfortable plan.

Since Dave and I were still on good terms and he was home all day, I asked him if I could stay with him while Ellen worked. I knew that it was not Dave's responsibility to alleviate my fears, but he was the only person who understood my predicament. For two months, I stayed with Dave while Ellen worked.

We were all traumatized by this muddled situation. Dave, suffering from depression and rejection, continued to drink too much. He and I got along fine when he was sober, but after several drinks his personality changed. Instead of being easy-going and glad to see me, he became morose and menacing. Sometimes he would stare at me with a hatred so intense I thought he might be capable of murder. My decision to move in with Ellen was the spark that ignited Dave's smoldering rage. He had been angry for years over the way his parents treated him and now he was moving deeper inside to a place where I could no longer reach him. I had hurt him deeply by going with Ellen and he was protecting himself by building an impenetrable wall around himself. I became even more sad and frightened for myself and the children, who divided their time between Dave and my parents.

The first of two truly frightening incidents occurred early in 1977. I needed to get something out of the house and called Dave to see if Ellen and I could come over. When we entered, Dave was waiting with a loaded double-barreled shotgun. Luckily, the boys were in school. He had been drinking but was still coherent and in control. He ordered us to sit on the couch while he stood across the room with the gun pointed at us. He kept telling us he could blow us away at any minute and would do so if either of us moved. Fearful that any sign of affection or fear would amplify his rage, Ellen and I avoided making eye contact. I knew the gun was loaded because he kept taking the shells in and out of the chamber. I told myself he was only bluffing, that he was incapable of killing someone, but he had a murderous look in his eyes. His angry stare and unpredictability frightened me. It also frightened me to know that he had planned this. He knew we were coming because I had called to tell him so. As I sat there, thinking of a way to escape, my mind was flooded by disturbing thoughts. I thought about the murders on the news that resulted from domestic violence. I thought about crimes of passion and saw myself as another statistic. Then I considered the killer who thinks, "If I can't have her, nobody can." I kept a conversation going, trying to defuse his anger. After forty-five minutes of being held hostage and trying to judge Dave's state of mind, I feigned serious illness which distracted him. I doubled over, pretending to be in serious pain. I said, "Dave, I need a doctor. I have to go to the emergency room." The three of us got into Ellen's car and she drove us to the hospital.

On arrival, I pulled a staff member aside and explained the situation. "I really don't need a doctor. My husband, who is here with me, was holding my friend and I hostage with a shotgun. I faked illness, hoping he'd fall for it so we could get to a safe place. Now that we're here, I don't know how you can help us."

The nurse said, "First, I need to take down your personal information, then I'll call the police." I sat on a bed in the emergency room, fearful and anxious. I dreaded talking to the police. When they arrived, we went into a private room to talk. Dave and Ellen were sitting in the waiting room. At the end of the interview, the cops asked if I wanted to press charges against Dave. I declined. I just couldn't do it. I blamed myself for the incident and Dave's state of mind.

The police took Dave home and confiscated his valuable gun collection. The fact that Dave was willing to put the gun down and ride to the hospital convinced me that he was bluffing. My feigned illness was a way for all of us to become gracefully disentangled.

After this incident, I was afraid to stay with Dave. I went back to my previous routine of sitting in the car in the hospital lot or sitting in the hospital lobby. I was lonely and despondent. My family was barely speaking to me and Ellen was still unaware that I couldn't be alone. I missed my sons, Robert and Stephen, who were ten and six, respectively. They were now spending most of their time with my parents. I felt terribly guilty leaving my sons with my parents, but at the time there were no other options that I could see. I was afraid I would panic if I was alone with them; they refused to stay overnight with me and Ellen; Dave, who was supposed to be caring for them, was spending most evenings out drinking. At a time when my sons should have been bonding with me and their father, they were bonding with my parents who kept telling them that Dave and I were losers and Ellen was an evil intruder. Until I could settle into a more stable and routine existence,

I saw no hope for a different relationship with any of them.

A few weeks after the gun crisis, Dave called to apologize for his out-of-control behavior. He encouraged me to return while Ellen worked, promising that everything would be fine. Since he sounded sane and sober over the phone and I was desperate to get away from the hospital routine, I agreed to return to our former arrangement. Everything went smoothly until the fourth week of my day-camp-like stay when another terrible incident occurred.

Early one afternoon, Dave was in the kitchen chopping vegetables and drinking beer. I was leaning on the kitchen counter conversing with him while he worked. What had begun as a normal conversation suddenly turned into a heated discussion about our strange living situation. I could tell by Dave's eyes that he was becoming enraged. I knew it was time for me to get out before he lost control. My car keys were lying on the counter close to me and as I reached to grab them, Dave slammed the heavy chopping knife down by my keys. The blade just missed my hand. I got my keys and ran, chased by Dave with the knife. I beat him to my car, got in and locked the doors. I backed out of the driveway with him frantically banging the knife on the windshield. Trembling, I drove to the hospital and paged Ellen. When she saw how shaken I was, she advised me to stay away from Dave's because he was not to be trusted. This would have been the perfect time to tell Ellen that I couldn't stay alone but I was not in the mood to have this discussion.

Now I was in a real bind because I couldn't face sitting in the hospital parking lot again. I had no idea how I was going to manage. I was depressed, isolated and terrified. My gynecologist, who had noticed but not pursued my high de-gree of anxiety, had given me a refillable Valium prescription. Though I rarely took the Valium, I decided that I needed something now to get me through Ellen's work day. It was my goal to stay pleasantly sedated but still functional. The Valium took just enough edge off my fear to allow me to drop Ellen at the hospital and return to her house alone. When I became frightened, I tried the distraction technique of keeping busy, but it was not as effective now as it had been when Dave worked at the florist shop and I was alone. Then, I knew that I could call Dave and he would come home. Since Ellen had no knowledge of my problem, it was point-less to call her at work. Even if I needed her to rescue me, she couldn't leave the hospital.

My daily survival strategy consisted of a small amount of Valium and forcing myself to take new risks. Though at times I still fell back on the refuge of the hospital parking lot and lobby, I was trying to spend increased time home alone. On days when I felt more anxious and didn't want to be alone or go to the hospital lot, I went to the public library where I spent hours reading. I found it helpful to be around other people in an impersonal setting where I could escape quickly and easily with no questions asked.

Every day was a struggle—something to be gotten through. Only when I picked Ellen up after work could I breathe with relief that I had made it through another day. If she asked me how my day went, I'd tell her nonchalantly that I cleaned house or went to the library. Because my activities seemed normal, she had no reason to question them. But I was running out of energy to maintain the illusion that I was an independent, functional person. It was time to be honest about my situation.

I approached Ellen on one of her days off from work. I was in the bedroom, sitting on the edge of the bed, when I called her into the room. I was terrified and didn't know how to begin my confession. Ellen sat down next to me and I started to cry. She said, "What's wrong? Are you upset with me about something? Whatever it is, you can tell me. You'll feel better if you talk about what's bothering you. Maybe I can help you."

By now I was sobbing so hard, I could only get the words out in short bursts. "There's something I've been wanting to tell you since we've been together. I was afraid if you knew the truth about me, you'd leave."

"Nothing can be bad enough for me to leave you. I love you. Please tell me what's wrong."

As I cried continuously, I told Ellen about my ten-year struggle with panic and anxiety. She was shocked that I had stayed in the car all day at the hospital. I enumerated the list of things I couldn't do: drive out of town alone, fly in a plane, stand in a store or bank line, be in crowds, stay home alone and on and on. I explained the feeling of terror that overcame me when I just thought about being in a feared situation. "That's why I've been staying at Dave's. He's the only person who knows about this problem. Dave has been my rock, my support person. His tolerance of my predicament has added to the guilt I feel about leaving him." I explained to Ellen the important role of the support person and how impossible it would be for me to function without one.

Ellen was as baffled as I about what was happening to me. In her many years of nursing, she had never heard of such a condition. The unknown nature of the problem did nothing to reassure me. It only reinforced my belief that the condition was specific to me. Even though Ellen had no medical knowledge about my panic situation, she lovingly agreed to be my support person. She said, "I'm so sorry you couldn't talk about this earlier. I would never leave you. I'm just sorry that you live in such a state of fear."

She held me close and said, "We'll fight this together. There must be someone out there who knows what you have and how to fix it. I'm sure you're not the only person with panic attacks. You must hang in there until we can find help."

Knowing I could no longer go back to Dave and hating the panicky feelings that were ruining my life, it was imperative that I find a way to go forward.

"What are we going to do?"

After the gun and knife incidents, my marriage to Dave was over. The trust between us had been breached by both of us and his anger frightened me. I still loved him and wished we had possessed the foresight and strength to make a different life for ourselves. Though I was terrified to make the permanent transition from Dave to Ellen, I couldn't live with one foot planted on either side of an ever-widening chasm. The thought of leaving Dave was so difficult that at times I fantasized about him, me and Ellen living together in some impossibly idyllic way.

To safely make the leap to Ellen, she and I needed a survival plan, one that would allow us to gain some control over our lives. Now that Ellen knew how difficult it was for me to be alone, she felt guilty going to work. She knew that I struggled to get through each day of staying alone, sitting in the hospital lot or spending time at the library. Since we didn't know how to alleviate my fear and I needed an income, what were we going to do? Ellen could support herself but how was I going to support myself? If I had to be close to Ellen, my support person, how could I possibly function in a job setting where I had no control? I had functioned well with Dave at the flower shop only because we were there together. The idea of going it alone was inconceivable. However strange the financial setup was with Dave, I never worried about the lack of money. When I left Dave permanently, I would be on my own financially.

It occurred to me to take over operation of the flower shop in Davis that Dave and I had purchased in 1972 and still owned. The store was being managed by the same designer since the time of our purchase. If Ellen and I took over the daily operation of the store, we could solve the two problems of making a living and being together. Ellen was skeptical. "I don't know anything about retail and I'm not real comfortable leaving the hospital. Nursing is grueling work, but I know I'll get a regular paycheck. On the other hand, it would be nice to work together and have more freedom."

I assured her it was workable. "Why don't we try? If it doesn't work out, I can sell the business. You'll be able to learn the basics quickly from me and the staff that is already in place. The designer-manager would stay on as the designer, I would manage the finances and you, who are good with people, could manage sales and personnel."

With Ellen and I agreeing to work together, I approached Dave about the business. Since he and I had already been discussing divorce, I offered to give up alimony in exchange for his share of the business. He agreed to this arrangement, making me sole owner of the business. At the end of 1977,

Ellen resigned from the hospital and we started working together in the flower shop.

We commuted every day to the store, located seven miles from our house. This was a manageable drive as long as Ellen and I were together. But I soon began obsessing on all the scenarios that might force us to be apart. To end my obsession, we adopted the same pattern of living that Dave and I had shared; we became inseparable. This meant we were never out of each other's sight! We ran every errand together and if either one of us became ill, we both stayed home. My main focus in life became the attempt to anticipate every situation that would require that I drop everything to be with Ellen. If I lost sight of her in our store, I'd stop working and dash out of the office to find her. If we became separated in the grocery store and I lost sight of her, I panicked. Once I could see her and we reconnected, I relaxed.

When I told Ellen how fearful I became when she was out of sight, she tried to reason with me. "I would never just leave you alone. If I'm out of sight, just stay put and I'll find you. Nothing bad is going to happen to you. You can always have me paged. Besides, there are people around who would help you in an emergency." Though I knew what she said was true, it didn't help. In fact, it did the opposite by drawing more attention to my fear and my inability to manage it.

After commuting for over a year, in an attempt to alleviate some of the anxiety, Ellen sold her condo in the spring of 1979 and we moved to Davis. The move made our lives easier in many ways. We could come home for lunch, drive to the business in ten minutes and feel like we were part of a more tolerant and progressive community. We were able to leave behind the Woodland gossips who knew my parents and delighted in talking about their *lesbian* daughter. One of these inveterate gossips actually parted cereal boxes to catch a glimpse of me and Ellen in the grocery store. With every sighting of the *lesbians*, she'd call my father with the same announcement, "I saw your daughter and her girlfriend in the grocery store today." Ellen's response to this was always, "Lesbians have to eat too."

I had hoped that the move would make it easier for me to stay home alone or come and go to the shop by myself. But no matter what I told myself or how hard I tried, nothing changed. I still needed to be with Ellen all the time. I was getting to the point where I didn't know how much longer I could go on living this way. In addition to being depressed and desperate, I blamed myself for the panicky feelings and for not being able to control them. I was stuck. I needed professional help but still didn't know where to find it.

Another part of the "What are we going to do?" question concerned my children. I knew that if I didn't step into their lives soon, I ran the risk of losing them forever. Now that Ellen and I were settled in a larger home and a more profitable business, I wanted the boys to move in with us, even though I questioned my ability to care for them. If I couldn't get through a day without being glued to Ellen, how could I provide a stable environment for them? How was I going to take them to school, to appointments, be home alone with them or take them on fun outings? From the time my children were born, the priority of finding ways to maneuver around my fear and anxiety had interfered with my ability to form an inviolable bond with them. Realistically, in order to care for the boys, I needed to be strong and independent enough to make them feel safe and secure. I didn't know how I could manage, but I missed my kids and was determined to fight for them.

After several days of ferocious phone battles with my parents, the boys moved in with us during the fall of 1979. Robert was twelve and Stephen was eight. While the boys were trying to adapt to new schools and a new environment, the battle with my parents raged on. Almost daily there was some form of grandparental interference. Often, it was an after school phone call from my mother asking Stephen if there was food in the house. One time, I listened in to a call from my mother. She was quizzing Stephen. "How do your mom and Ellen treat you and your brother? Does your mother cook dinner? Do you get your homework done?" When Stephen started crying, my mother said, "Don't worry. Just be patient. Your grandfather and I will get you out of there as soon as we can."

One day, without notifying me, my mother picked Stephen up from school and took him to McDonald's. When Ellen and I arrived at the school, Stephen was already gone. When I rushed into the principal's office seeking Stephen's whereabouts, her response was, "His grandmother picked him up. Didn't you know?" The critical tone of her voice forced me to explain the details of the ongoing battle between me and my parents. Horrified, she offered to tell my parents that they weren't authorized to pick him up without my permission. But, I declined. I wanted to try to have a reasonable discussion with them without escalating the battle by calling in enforcers. Unfortunately, trying to have a reasonable discussion with them was impossible. When I tried to put rules in place, they dug in deeper, more determined than ever to rescue the kids.

Dave was no help. He had given me custody of the children and rarely saw them. It would've been nice to have had an emotionally strong man to help me fight the enemy, but Dave wasn't present. His parents didn't approve of the boys living with me, but they stayed off the battlefield.

Ellen tried to help, but came across as defensive and angry. She'd say, "I feel like we're under constant attack and this makes me mad. I know the kids resent me. They see me as the intruder who broke up their family. How can they accept us when we've been portrayed as evil people? Every time I try to help Stephen with his homework, he cries. Robert, who never brings any work home, would never accept help from me. I feel badly for the kids. With all this turmoil in their lives, how can they possibly function well in school?"

My parents' constant interference created an environment of instability and anxiety. Instead of trying to support the boys and us in a positive way, they did everything possible to undermine us. My father went as far as threatening to sue me for custody of the boys. In response, Ellen became defensive and I became passive and withdrawn, which further sabotaged my ability to establish a positive relationship with my children.

Diagnosis and Therapy

I first heard the word *agoraphobia* in 1983. I had been referred to Scripps Clinic in La Jolla by my allergist who wanted another opinion about my recent run of upper respiratory infections. La Jolla is near San Diego, about a ten-hour drive south from my home. After the Santa Barbara ordeal with Dave back in 1967, driving was not an option. The only good alternative was to fly. After making the clinic appointment and purchasing the airline tickets, I started obsessing on everything that could go wrong. *What if the plane crashes? What if something happens to Ellen while we're there and I have to manage by myself? What if I hyperventilate on the plane and make a fool of myself? What if I need to get off the plane?* When the time came to leave, I could board the plane only after taking several Valium.

We arrived safely but instead of being relieved, I began obsessing about the trip home. Since the scheduled medical workup lasted five days, we stayed in La Jolla for a week. When I wasn't at the clinic, I tried to enjoy the amazing beauty of La Jolla, which sits nestled in a cove of the Pacific

Ocean. I hoped that the beauty and sound of the waves would calm my mind but they were no match for the intrusive and frightening thoughts about the flight home.

The five days at the clinic were almost as frightening and annoying as my obsessing on flying. Every day was filled with tests and consultations. I was assigned a primary physician, an allergist, who was responsible for determining what tests I would have and what other physicians would participate in the evaluation. Every morning when I arrived, I checked in with my primary physician to get my lab slips and instructions for the day. When I met with my doctor on the third day, he commented on my anxiety and depression. He referred me to a staff psychiatrist. In a tearful consultation, I told the psychiatrist about my panicky feelings, my inability to be home alone, my fear of hyperventilating and my inability to function without a support person. Very routinely and with no hesitation, he told me I had agoraphobia. I looked at him quizzically, waiting for an explanation of the diagnosis he had just delivered, but he didn't elaborate on it. Instead, he suggested I find a therapist in my area who specialized in treating agoraphobia. While I was grateful for the diagnosis, I was stymied by the lack of helpful information. If I couldn't rely on a respected professional to provide information or a source for help, I doubted my ability to find it on my own.

I returned to my primary physician at the clinic for a summary report of my tests and exams. When the doctor read the psychiatrist's diagnosis aloud, he joked about agoraphobia being the fear of agriculture. I realized he didn't have the slightest idea about the meaning of agoraphobia or the role it played in my ongoing state of anxiety and depression. I left the clinic frustrated with the lack of information about agoraphobia, but I was relieved to know that the life-altering feelings I was experiencing had a name.

When I returned home, I enthusiastically searched the local book stores for information on agoraphobia. I found nothing. I resorted to the dictionary which defined agoraphobia as "an abnormal fear of being in open or public places." Because this definition didn't describe the kind of fear I was experiencing, I thought the psychiatrist had made a diagnostic error. Unable to find any information on this condition, it seemed futile to look for a professional who could treat it. Again discouraged, I continued the business of living around my fears.

The year I went to Scripps Clinic was also the year Stephen moved in with my parents. Robert stayed with me and Ellen. He was in high school and didn't want to leave his friends. Stephen was in junior high and miserable. He was being teased mercilessly by a group of junior high boys. The tormentors shoved him off his bike, hid in bushes and ambushed him, called him a "fag," and made fun of him for living with lesbians. They egged our house and car and spray-painted "queer" on our garage door. When these attacks became more frequent, Stephen was afraid to go to school. He cried and begged to move to his grandparents'. When I saw how frightened and depressed he was, I had to let him go, even though I felt like I was feeding him to the wolves.

Because the schools in Davis were considered excellent, Stephen remained in the same junior high with the bullies, who fortunately had now moved on to other targets. My parents drove him the seven miles to and from school. The teachers and counseling staff were aware that I lived with Ellen and that Stephen lived with his grandparents. When there were problems, the school called me. Soon after Stephen had moved, I was summoned to a lengthy conference with his teachers, the school psychologist and the counselors. There were two problems they wanted to discuss. The first was my father, who kept calling the school to offer his unsolicited opinions and to badger the staff for information about Stephen. The second was Stephen. The staff was concerned about him because he seemed listless and depressed. They wanted to know why Stephen had moved to his grandparents'. After I explained the history of the grandparent ordeal, the school psychologist advised me to find a family therapist who could intercede and help sort out this destructive family dynamic.

Ellen and I found Barbara, a kind, compassionate middle-aged therapist whom we liked immediately. The plan was for Ellen and me to see her first to provide background information; then she'd see my sons, both separately and together. Ultimately, the extended family would join the sessions. Those who would be involved included me and Ellen, my parents, the boys and Dave. The goal of the family sessions was for everyone to be heard so we could resolve our differences. The sessions with Ellen and me went well, but my sons refused to see the therapist. When I was able to coax them into her office, they wouldn't talk.

When it was time for the family sessions, Barbara included one of her male colleagues who specialized in group family therapy. Everyone named above attended the first session. I had explained the school situation to Dave, pleading with him to attend the meetings. The outcome of the sessions was heralded by the atmosphere in the therapists' waiting room. My sons sat with my parents, while Dave sat with me and Ellen. There was no eye contact and nobody spoke. With no hint of communication or compatibility, it was clear we were facing an impasse.

At the beginning of the first session, the therapists explained the rules of engagement and the purpose of the meetings. The purpose, of course, was for everyone to be able to share their feelings and concerns in a safe place and to establish methods that would enable better understanding and dialogue. The discussions were to be centered around the welfare of the children. When the therapists began by describing the situation as they understood it, my father interrupted to announce his point of view. "The boys are screwed up because Dave and my daughter are terrible parents. What kind of mother deserts her family to be with an overbearing lesbian? Their grandparents are the only ones concerned about them."

The therapists tried to maintain order by telling him to wait his turn to speak. This made him furious, while my mother remained silent and passive. At the end of the session, he announced he wasn't coming back. By the following week, though, he had changed his mind.

During the second session, whenever anyone, including the therapists, tried to speak, my father interrupted. He leaped up to say, "I don't have to sit and listen to this bullshit. I don't need other people telling me how to run my life. When I leave today, I'm not coming back." Though both therapists were competent, the session had spun out of control. Under the circumstances, nothing important could be accomplished. We were all glad when the session ended and we parted ways.

Trying to have a rational discussion with my father was hopeless. While Ellen, Dave and I had come to the sessions hoping to express our concerns and feelings, my father had squandered the opportunity for achieving any meaningful contact or resolution.

Feeling beaten down and discouraged by the outcome of the meetings, Ellen and I continued to see Barbara. After seeing my father's performance, she had a clear idea of the insanity we were dealing with. We saw her separately and together for two years. The focus of our therapy was the painful examination of our childhoods. The purpose of this examination was to help us understand the past and its impact on our adult lives. Another focus of our work was learning how to establish boundaries. Barbara recognized that I was intimidated by my father, making me vulnerable and incapable of protecting myself and my children. She taught me how to be more assertive by drawing protective boundaries designed to mitigate my father's power and interference.

About eight months after I started therapy, I began responding differently to my father. For example, I told him that whatever happened with my sons at school was none of his business. I was their mother and I would deal with the school. I asked the school staff to ignore my father if he called or showed up. When he realized he could no longer intimidate me, he blamed the therapist for brainwashing me and turning me against him. He got so angry, he went to Barbara's office, which was in her house. When she answered the door, he verbally attacked her by threatening to have her license revoked for giving bad advice. The next time I saw her she told me about the incident and how shaken she was by it. She warned him that she'd call the police if he ever came back. When I told her about the new approach I had taken, she reasoned that setting boundaries for him had threatened his power and that he saw the therapist as a threat and an instigator. To counter this, he used the only tactic he understood, which was to threaten her.

During the two years I spent in therapy, I addressed my panicky feelings and the Scripps psychiatrist's diagnosis of agoraphobia. I was hoping Barbara could help me with this specific problem but at that time it was beyond her scope of knowledge. She recommended that I continue my search for reading material and for a therapist who specialized in treating agoraphobia.

By 1985, I was tired and ready to discontinue my therapy. Though I still didn't understand the meaning of the word agoraphobia, Barbara had helped me begin the process of working systematically through my childhood to find clues that might have contributed to the development of my fear and anxiety. When I found meaningful clues, she had advised that in addition to being intellectually aware of them, it was important to write them down and to be aware of how they made me feel. She had assured me that with introspection, time and determination, the pieces would come together and I would see the whole picture.

PART FOUR
Moving Forward
1987 and Beyond

The Chorus

When Ellen volunteered to direct a women's chorus in the spring of 1987, I was still trying to get up the nerve to find an appropriate therapist. The chorus practiced weekly in Sacramento. I felt angry about her commitment to this endeavor, yet I had encouraged her to become the director for two reasons: she is an excellent musician who needed a musical outlet, and I felt guilty about the sacrifices she had made and the restrictions she had endured to function as my support person. Ellen knew I was angry about the chorus, but was determined to participate in spite of my anger and fear. She said, "You can come with me or stay home. If you don't want to sing, then bring a book or your earphones. I've been isolated because you can't go anywhere, and I need socialization. I'm sorry this is so hard for you, but it's important to me. You'll be all right." The chorus met on Monday evenings in a church in one of the oldest, most crime-ridden areas of the city. I panicked just thinking about staying home alone. Since going with Ellen was the lesser of the fears, I trudged ungraciously to chorus every Monday evening.

At first, I just sat off by myself, angry, sullen and aloof. I was mad at Ellen for enjoying something that made me so uncomfortable and even angrier at myself for not being able to stay home alone. After weeks of isolating myself in an unfriendly manner, I decided to join the chorus. I'm ashamed to confess that even though I loved music, I joined out of fear. I envisioned future performances involving staging that might relegate me to some distant, isolated rehearsal room in a strange building while Ellen was on stage and out of reach. If I became a participant, I would never be far away from Ellen.

As time went on, many of my fears began to intensify and coalesce in the chorus experience. By participating in the chorus, I was unwittingly subjected to many fear-provoking situations. There were always concerts being planned and as soon as a new concert date was announced, I began to dread that day's arrival. I pictured performances in large buildings where parking might be distant, scary and inconvenient. I feared being separated from Ellen in the crush of a crowd. I spent weeks before every concert imagining all the frightening things that could go wrong and worrying about how I would cope with the variety of potential threats. While I was frightened and morose, the other members bubbled with an energy and enthusiasm that only served to amplify my misery.

As the director, Ellen was responsible for choosing and obtaining the music. Locally, choral sheet music was scarce, but Ellen found a place in San Francisco that carried a large selection. Prior to our first trip there, I spent days imagining frightening scenarios. I was convinced that on the very day we chose to go, the largest earthquake in history would hit San Francisco and we'd be buried half-alive in a pile of rubble or left stranded in the city. Perhaps Ellen might be killed and I would be left alone with no escape until the roads and bridges were repaired. Worse yet, the quake could strike as we were crossing the Bay Bridge and we'd be hurled like dolls in toy cars into the icy waters, then eaten by sharks. When I tired of obsessing on a potential quake, my mind jumped to picturing the music store in an undesirable location with parking that necessitated walking many unsafe blocks lined with menacing characters. I wished I could stay home alone and leave Ellen to the tasks that were so enjoyable to her. Needless to say, my dire obsessions dampened her enthusiasm.

Unable to keep my fears to myself, I vocalized them. I wanted Ellen to understand how frightened I was and to offer some consolation. Like a child, I pummeled Ellen with questions. "Why do we have to go to San Francisco for music? Can't you find something in Sacramento? It seems unreasonable to drive so far in lots of traffic just for music. What if the store is in a bad part of town or we can't find parking? Can't we put this trip off?"

Ellen lost patience with me and said, "Why does everything have to be an ordeal? Can't you ever just get in the car and go? People drive to San Francisco all the time and nothing happens to them. I'm sure we'll find parking. While I shop, you can distract yourself with a book. Before you know it, we'll be back home. If you'd quit dwelling on everything that could go wrong, you'd feel much better." When Ellen talked to me this way, I felt lonely and misunderstood, like the only person living with panic and fear.

On the morning we left for San Francisco, I fortified myself with Valium. Having failed to encounter an earthquake (so far), we located the music store in one of the seediest areas of town, exactly as I'd envisioned: boarded-up businesses and scary-looking men leaning in doorways. I was terrified. My heart raced, my throat tightened and I started to cry. I begged Ellen to shop for music elsewhere, but she insisted on going inside.

The store was on the third floor of a decrepit building. We were greeted by a creaky old elevator that I could hear clanking its way down the shaft. I decided to check out the stairs, but the dark, isolated stairwell made the elevator more appealing. I tried to console myself with the fact that the employees in the building used the elevator daily and that elevators were supposed to undergo periodic maintenance checks.

When the doors opened onto the third floor, I expected to find a ghoulish proprietor sitting behind a counter waiting to ensnare us. Instead, the large room was buzzing with normal-looking customers and employees. While Ellen spent four hours shopping for music, I spent the entire time trying not to hyperventilate. I tried to distract myself by reading a book or looking at music but I was so tense that it was an effort to breathe, swallow and hold back tears. I felt like Dorothy in Oz; I just wanted to be home. During the four hours we spent in the store, not one rational thought crossed my mind. The possibilities for disaster immediately crowded out any positive thought that might have improved the day.

After the San Francisco trip, I developed a new and unreasonable disdain for everything relating to the chorus. To mitigate my high level of fear, I also began to develop strict criteria and control over issues that Ellen found irrelevant and inane. For example, due to the threatening neighborhood where we practiced, I insisted on leaving home early enough to park immediately in front of the rehearsal door. When we didn't arrive in time to park in a certain "safe" place, I became angry and sulked through rehearsal. Once we were in the rehearsal room, every time the door opened, I was afraid that a psychopath or an armed addict in need of money was coming in to steal our purses or murder us. My own fears wouldn't allow me to understand why any rational person would join a chorus that practiced in the neighborhood with the highest crime rate in the city. I kept hoping everyone would quit so I could stay home in my safe environment.

In addition to my endless obsession over criteria concerning the chorus, I was surprised by a feeling of latent homophobia that had surfaced. I knew that the majority of members were lesbians, but I didn't feel comfortable with them or the lesbian label that came with membership. These feelings reignited the conflict I had about my sexual orientation: I wanted to be with Ellen, but I missed men in general and Dave in particular. With fear and conflict tormenting me, there were days when I felt like I didn't fit in anywhere or with anyone.

Regardless of how I felt, I knew Ellen enjoyed directing and was not going to quit just because I was paranoid and miserable. My anger toward the chorus stemmed from being forced, in spite of my fears, to leave my comfort zone. I couldn't continue living this way; something positive and constructive had to happen. Though I knew I needed help, I was still reluctant to pursue therapy for my agoraphobia; I was afraid of what I might have to go through to get better.

Ohio and Disney World

In the early summer of 1987, Ellen received an invitation to her high school reunion in Columbus, Ohio. Ellen, excited about the reunion, kept mentioning her desire to attend. I cringed whenever she said, "I'd love to go to my reunion. I haven't seen my friends in years and I miss them. If I went home, I could visit my mother. I'd like you to meet my classmates and see where I grew up. I know way more about your family and friends than you do about mine. I really want you to come with me."

As I listened to Ellen's excitement and hopefulness, I felt guilty and trapped: guilty for being an impediment and trapped by a decision I didn't want to make. Believing I had been challenged beyond my capacities by the chorus experience, I couldn't imagine making a trip to Ohio. When Ellen told me she was making plans to go with or without me, I looked at her as if she'd gone insane. "You must be kidding. My tolerance level has already been stretched thin by the chorus. How do you expect me to fly to Ohio? I know you've put up with my panic problem for years and

166

you really want to go to your reunion, but the idea of this trip is unreasonable and way beyond terrifying. I simply can't go."

Ellen responded, "I know this is a lot to ask, but the reunion is important to me. You feel safe with me and you'll be fine. You can take Valium for the plane ride and once we're settled there, we'll have fun. I know you can do this even if you think you can't."

There was no good way to respond to the situation. Ellen was going with or without me and I had to choose between two frightening alternatives: going with her or staying home alone. I chose to go. But anticipating the trip filled me with so much horror that I hoped I would become gravely ill or die as a way out. While Ellen and I were planning our trip, my younger son informed me that he and my mother were going to Disney World in August. The idea arose that it would be nice if the four of us could meet in Florida, tour Disney World and Epcot Center, then fly home together. Ellen and I agreed to this plan. The thought of meeting my son and mother and flying home with them gave me a sense of security. If something went wrong, there would be four of us to deal with it instead of two.

When it came time to leave home, I was exhausted from obsessing about the trip. I took my Valium and resigned myself to fate. At least Ellen and I would die together if the plane went down.

We landed safely in Columbus. The plan was to spend five days there then fly to Florida. Ellen was excited about introducing me to her classmates and when I could relax, usually after a swim or some wine, I enjoyed myself. But lurking beneath my enjoyment was the fear of getting back onto a plane. I kept telling myself that the flight from Columbus to Orlando was much shorter than the flight from California to Ohio and if I could survive one flight, I could do it again. Besides, my son and mother would be waiting for us in Florida.

It was suffocatingly hot and humid when we stepped off the plane in Orlando. There were tourists everywhere. We took a shuttle to our hotel, one of many pastel, stuccoed hotels inhabited by exuberant theme-park bound guests. Though our hotel was making an attempt to come across as elegant and sophisticated, the décor screamed phony and corny. Because of the humidity, the entire hotel emanated a musty smell that permeated the atmosphere. Everything had a Disney theme. There were Cinderella chandeliers, Goofy wastebaskets and at dinner, I expected Mickey to jump onto the table singing *It's a Small World*. I was tired of Disney World before I even got to the park.

The park was jammed. Rather than stand in long lines waiting for the popular rides, Ellen and I went on the boring, educational rides. Most days we separated from my son and mother, meeting up at designated locations throughout the day. By the end of the third day, I was beginning to find the entire Disney experience cloying and claustrophobic. We were scheduled to depart on day six and I could hardly wait to leave.

On the day of departure, we awoke to hurricane force winds. The palm trees on the hotel grounds were leaning parallel to the ground, the pool water was sloshing around and all the deck chairs were being tossed by the wind.

I told Ellen, "There's no way I'm flying in this weather. How can a plane even take off in this wind? Please call the airport and change our reservations. Maybe the wind will be calmer tomorrow. Ask the people at airport reservations if the plane is really taking off."

Ellen replied, "I'll try to change the reservations, but I doubt the weather will be any different tomorrow. The pilots and airlines know what they're doing. They don't let planes fly in unsafe conditions. But, I'll call and see what they say." There was no problem changing our flight to the next day, but the airline warned Ellen that the weather would likely be the same. And, yes, they said, planes do take off safely in windy conditions.

I stayed awake most of the night waiting for the wind to stop, but nothing changed. Since there were no plane crashes on the news, reason told me that the plane we were supposed to be on the previous day had taken off and landed safely. Now, I wished I had left yesterday. I'd be home now and not here facing the same problem.

While boarding our new flight, I felt my hands getting clammy and my breathing becoming more shallow, in spite of the ten milligrams of Valium I'd swallowed. To keep from hyperventilating, I tried to focus on the boarding passengers instead of myself. Ellen and I were seated across the aisle and three rows back from my son and mother. They were talking and laughing while I was trying to look and feel normal.

As the plane backed away from the terminal, a loud metallic clank startled everyone. It sounded as if some integral part of the plane had fallen off. The pilot pulled the plane back into the loading area of the terminal as the stewardess announced, "The plane has encountered a mechanical problem. It's nothing serious, but we'll be grounded for a while. I'll keep you informed of our estimated departure. Everyone must remain in their seats." I couldn't believe this was happening; first, the wild wind and now a mechanical problem.

After forty-five minutes of sitting in a stuffy cabin with no sign of movement, I panicked. I cried and screamed, "I have to get off this plane. Now!! I'm hyperventilating and I need to get out." Ellen advised me to take more Valium. She tried to calm me by insisting we'd be on our way soon. The stewardess rushed over and asked if she could help. She brought water so I could take the Valium but I insisted on getting off the plane. As the other passengers stared at me, I shouted, "Quit staring, you morons! I have a problem and I need to get out of here." People looked at me like I was nuts. My son and mother ignored me.

The stewardess returned to my seat and said, "It is against protocol to let passengers off the plane after boarding, but we will make an exception for you. The captain will let you wait in the passenger boarding area in the terminal until the plane is ready." I explained that Ellen had to accompany me because I couldn't get off the plane without her. This caused another hassle, but the captain let her off with me.

Ellen and I sat alone in the deserted terminal. I sobbed and sobbed. "I can't get back on that plane. There's something wrong with it. I want to take a bus or a train home."

She tried to reason with me. "We're not taking a bus or a train; at least I'm not. After three days on either of those you'd be glad to be on a plane. Besides, our luggage is on the plane. You'll be fine! Just trust that the airline will fix the problem and we'll be home by this evening."

When the stewardess came out to check on us and saw me crying, she said, "There's someone on the plane who wants to talk to you. Maybe he can help you feel better." A minute later, the captain came out. He introduced himself and asked me to follow him into the cockpit. Shakily, I did so. As I stood behind his seat, he introduced me to the co-pilot and explained the function of some of the numerous lights and switches that seemed to engulf the cramped cockpit. When I calmed down, he looked at me very seriously. "I hear you're having a hard time being on a plane and that you're frightened by the sound you heard. I want you to know that I've been a pilot for many years and have been responsible for thousands of lives. I would never fly a plane that was unsafe. Just like my passengers, I want to get home safely. I have a wife and three children who I want to see again. I've flown all over the country for years and I always make it home. I'm sorry you're having such a hard time, but you must trust that I'll get you home safely. In a few minutes, we'll be ready for takeoff. You and your friend can return to your seats. If you start getting scared, remember what I've told you."

When I went back to my seat, I felt more calm and trusting. Through the remainder of the flight as the plane bumped through the air, I soothed myself by picturing the captain and repeating his calming words. I felt like

171

I had a real friend on board, someone who cared how I felt. I've never forgotten the captain or his powerful act of kindness. I practically kissed the ground when we disembarked, but looking back at the plane and the small cockpit windows, I wished I could have thanked the captain one more time.

Therapy 1987:
Emerging From the Quicksand

After my embarrassing, out-of-control behavior on the plane, I could no longer put off finding a therapist. In a book I was reading about panic attacks and phobias, there was mention of a family therapist in Sacramento who specialized in treating panic disorder. I wrote down his name, looked up his phone number and stared at the information for a week, trying to get up the nerve to call. When I finally made the call, I told Mr. Roberts how frightened I was about making an appointment. To spare me the stress of coming to Sacramento for an initial meeting, he offered to drive to the flower shop and meet in my office. He said, "That way we can meet in a place where you feel comfortable. I will give you an overview of my approach to treatment. If you decide to work with me, we can set up a weekly meeting at my office."

On the day of our appointment, I awoke anxious and terrified, wondering why I had agreed to the meeting.

But when the therapist came into the office, my fear was allayed by his calm, kind and self-assured demeanor. His offer to meet me in my office indicated that he understood and empathized with my fear. During the meeting, he explained that he was a family therapist with a focus on behavioral modification, an approach to psychology which focuses on changing self-defeating behaviors. He gave me written information outlining his treatment plan, which included weekly therapy sessions, learning and practicing positive behaviors and listening to audio tapes. Though I was afraid of the work I might have to do, I committed to weekly appointments. I introduced him to Ellen, who as my partner and support person would be riding with me to the appointments.

On the way to my first appointment, I wanted to turn around, go home and ignore my commitment. Though I wanted help, I was angry that I had a problem I couldn't overcome by myself. In addition, after spending twenty years with nobody to help me, I wondered whether help was really available and if I had chosen the right therapist.

During my first two sessions with him, I described my family history, my first panic attack and the nature of my ongoing experience with panic and anxiety. His diagnosis: panic disorder with agoraphobia. He made a distinction between panic attacks with and without agoraphobia. "It is possible to have panic attacks without agoraphobia if there is no avoidance behavior. Since you avoid places where you fear having a panic attack, the diagnosis becomes panic attacks with agoraphobia."

He explained that I possessed an anxious personality and that the years of accumulated stress during my formative years, along with a probable genetic tendency toward anxiety and panic, set the stage for the development of panic disorder. My miscarriage and the months of unresolved bleeding were probably the events that pushed me over the edge into hyperventilation, a panic attack, and into the panic cycle. Using the events of my first panic attack in Santa Barbara as an example, he explained how the anxiety/panic cycle works.

While driving on the curvy roads, I became slightly nauseated, a not uncommon reaction to driving on winding roads. My intense focus on the nausea produced fear, which caused my body to release adrenaline. As my fear increased, my body produced more adrenaline, causing me to hyperventilate and panic. The feelings of nausea I experienced so intensely in the car, though not life-threatening or dangerous, produced enough fear and adrenaline to trigger the fight or flight response, a complex protective defense which prepares the body to fight or flee from real or perceived danger. In this instance, my brain was reacting to "perceived" danger, which produced the same adrenaline response as real danger. Because I didn't understand what had happened to me in Santa Barbara, when I returned home I began to anticipate and worry about being caught in the same fear-producing cycle in other situations. Eventually, as this negative anticipation spread, I began to avoid more places where I feared that I would hyperventilate and panic. This anxiety/panic cycle led to the development of panic disorder and agoraphobia.

Though intellectually I knew that most places and circumstances were as innocuous as inanimate objects, it didn't matter. What I feared was the anticipation of a panic attack and the frightening feeling of hyperventilation. Even when a panic attack subsided, I feared another attack was imminent. This meant that my brain was repeatedly reacting to perceived danger.

When my therapist and I re-examined my first panic attack in the light of this information, I realized that the catalyst for panic was the unchecked, distorted dialogue in my head about my body's response to perceived threats. The focus of my therapy would be learning to control or avert panic attacks by changing my behavior and the negative messages I was sending to my brain.

New Challenges

Tuning in to My Body

My first lesson focused on the role that anxiety plays in the development and perpetuation of panic disorder. Before I could begin to practice desensitizing myself to the situations that triggered panic, I had to learn how to monitor and decrease my anxiety. My therapist gave me an audio tape to listen to several times a day. He had produced and recorded the tape which focused on relaxation and breathing techniques designed to reduce anxiety. Prior to therapy, I had been unaware of the tension in my body. Though I lived in a state of tension and hypervigilance, always braced for some disaster or the next panic attack, I had never given this way of being a second thought. Since anxiety had become my normal state, learning to relax wasn't easy. When I first started listening to the tape, the feeling of calm lasted only as long as the twenty-minute tape. Now that I knew how much lighter and calmer I felt when the tension left for those twenty minutes, I wanted the relaxed feeling to continue throughout the day. But lengthening the time of relaxation would require that in addition to listening to the tape, I learn to pay close attention to my body.

Developing the ability to scan my body for signs of tension took great effort. It was easy to go through the day thinking I was relaxed until I noticed that my teeth were clenched, I felt overwhelmed, my neck ached or some other sign of tension appeared. If I happened to notice any feelings of anxiety, I had a clue that I was tense. But if I didn't notice the signs of stress, I could go through an entire day in a knot. Since relaxation and tension are mutually exclusive, I knew that my recovery hinged on my ability to lower my level of anxiety. Though I knew I couldn't control the stress in my body without recognizing it, I didn't like focusing on my body. I associated my tendency to hyperventilate with paying too much attention to my body and my breathing. It wasn't until I learned that in order to control hyperventilation, I had to become aware of my breathing in a new and positive way.

One of Mr. Roberts's tapes focused on the importance of using abdominal breathing to diffuse panic and alleviate anxiety. In stressful situations, I found myself breathing rapidly from high in my chest. If the rapid and shallow breathing continued unchecked, the creeping tingling of hyperventilation began its ascent up my limbs. When I consciously shifted my breathing from my chest to my abdomen, the tingling diminished and the feeling of control increased. It became my goal to master the spontaneous transition from chest breathing to abdominal breathing.

After two weeks of listening to the breathing and relaxation tapes at least four times a day, I began to feel lighter as the tension in my body eased. I didn't startle as quickly and my temperament became more level. If I listened to a tape at bedtime, I rested better. I was beginning to feel less frantic and realized that this was probably the first time in years I had been this relaxed. As I became more relaxed, the panicky feelings associated with fearful thoughts loosened their grip on me. I developed a new awareness of how my body responds to fear and anxiety. This awareness made it possible for me to begin to change. As long as I continued to believe that panic attacks were caused by exterior situations such as driving or staying home alone, I remained a victim. The embryonic control I was beginning to feel increased my self-esteem and motivated me to face the next challenge.

Changing Negative Thoughts and Negative Self-Talk

The next step toward recovery was learning to become aware of the content of the on-going dialogue in my head: my self-talk. Like my breathing, my thoughts were automatic and I didn't question their content. Because they were so automatic, it took tremendous effort to really hear the messages that were repeated over and over. When I started paying attention to my interior dialogue, I was shocked by the frightening and demoralizing messages I found there.

Many days on awakening, I would begin the day by thinking, *What if something should happen today that would force me to be alone? How could I possibly survive alone? What if Ellen needs major surgery? I would have to sleep in a chair in the hospital because I couldn't be home alone. I would never be able to manage the business by myself.* Then I would tell myself, *My agoraphobia really gets me down. I'm never going to get better.* At the end of most days I was exhausted and depressed, but I was beginning to realize that my thoughts were directly affecting my perceptions and feelings.

With the negative interior dialogue replaying automatically in my head every day, it was impossible for me to have a calm, positive outlook on life. My negative thoughts were examples of distorted thinking which caused me to have a distorted, irrational view of reality. My distorted thinking took many forms but the end result was always the same: I felt frightened, defeated and depressed.

My homework for this part of therapy was to learn to pay attention to my self-talk, recognize the distorted thoughts and correct them with rational thoughts. For example, if I caught myself thinking, *If Ellen had to have surgery, I wouldn't be able to function on my own,* a rational counter to that thought might be: *If Ellen had surgery, I could manage. I could ask a friend for help or I would figure out how to manage on my own. I am a resourceful person. Besides, I am fortune telling. I am predicting and stressing over an event that may never happen.* Though my therapist was teaching me ways to counter the negative dialogue, the challenge was catching myself in the act. Sometimes days of negative talk would pass before I noticed. But like any other kind of practice, the more attention I paid to my thoughts, the less time it took to notice them.

Since positive thinking was not one of my strengths, to say the least, I created a generic positive retort that would cover most negative thoughts: *The chances of that particular event happening today are very slim. I don't want to waste energy on hypothetical situations. I need my energy for the present. If such a thing happens, I will be able to cope with it in the manner I choose.*

Even though I didn't really believe my positive, rational replacement thoughts, I made the effort to identify and challenge my negative self-talk at every opportunity. As I became more skilled at changing the negative talk to positive, I became more confident and less depressed. Sometimes on good days, I even believed the positive messages.

I moved through the prescribed mental exercises at my own pace. Sometimes, I could grasp and implement an exercise in one to two weeks, and other times it took longer. With every lesson building on the previous one, weekly therapy afforded me the opportunity to work through problems that impeded my progress. It was important to have a solid foundation before I moved on to more difficult challenges. Achieving that foundation took about two months.

Taking The First Big Step-Staying Home Alone

As I did my homework and practiced the new relaxation and breathing skills, I was aware that every lesson was preparing me to confront the situations I had carefully avoided for more than twenty years. Though I was armed with new knowledge and coping skills, I cringed at the thought of actually facing the situations that terrified me. My thoughts wandered into the big picture of me driving miles alone on the freeway, flying in planes and Ellen disappearing for hours to enjoy her new freedom. Such wild wanderings into a big, unknowable future only increased my anxiety, making the idea of change more threatening.

When I felt threatened and discouraged by the challenges ahead of me, Ellen was always there to cheer me on and to keep me focused on recovery.

Before I could start practicing new behaviors, I had to prioritize my goals and clearly define a course of action. My first two goals were to stay home alone while Ellen remained at work or ran errands, and to be able to drive around town by myself. The therapist and I worked together to develop a practice strategy that would gently move me forward. My plan was to work first on staying home alone for very short periods, gradually increasing the time as I became more comfortable. I was to begin by staying alone for five minutes three to four times a week. To maintain my resolve to practice, I could think only in terms of taking very small steps.

During the first week of practice, I stayed home alone for five minutes while Ellen drove around the block. As she drove away, I stood anxiously by the door and watched the car disappear. While standing alone in the house, my heart began racing and a lump began forming in my throat. I doubted my ability to survive for five minutes. For distraction, I turned the TV on and off and tried to read a magazine. I was too agitated to breathe abdominally or use my relaxation techniques. When I thought I couldn't take another minute of anxiety, Ellen pulled into the driveway. My high level of anxiety made me wonder if I had the fortitude to continue practicing.

Because I saw my therapist weekly, he was able to help me cope with the discouragement and frustration that sapped my energy and motivation. I needed a lot of support and encouragement and he and Ellen provided it. As I continued to practice, I learned that to sustain my commitment, I had to start managing my practice time in a more positive way.

Developing Survival Skills

After a few months of gradually increasing my time home alone by five-minute increments, I made it to thirty minutes. In a typical thirty-minute practice session, Ellen drove to the grocery store a few blocks from home. Before she left, I wrote down the store's phone number just in case I needed to have her paged; I needed the security of being able to get in touch with her. Nobody had cell phones in 1987.

As soon as Ellen stepped out the front door and I heard the car drive away, the negative self-talk began. *I am alone now. What if I pass out? There is no one here to help me. What if I call Ellen at the store and she's not there? I don't think I can stand this for thirty minutes.* After a few seconds of this talk, I recognized it and could feel how much it was frightening me. I practiced countering the negative messages with something more positive. *I am alone now but I can manage. I am perfectly capable of taking care of myself. I can distract myself in a number of ways. The chances of passing out are slim because I know how to control my breathing to prevent hyperventilation. I trust Ellen. If she says she is going to the store, she will be there.*

Though it took a great deal of focus and energy, I had to challenge every negative thought that entered my awareness. At first, every time Ellen left I bombarded myself with negative thoughts. When I became more adept at recognizing and challenging them, their impact and frequency diminished.

In addition to the mental invasion of the negative thoughts, I still experienced many of the physical reactions to fear: racing heart, sweaty palms, shallow breathing and a constrictive lump in my throat. To quell the physical sensations, I used distraction. I flipped through the TV channels, played the piano or cleaned the house. When I stayed distracted by motion, the physical sensations abated because I stopped focusing on my body. Though I was frustrated by not being able to focus at length on a singular project while at home, a few years later I would be relaxed enough to read, paint or actually fall asleep.

Two other forms of self-sabotage interfered significantly with my ability to practice staying home alone: berating myself for the things I couldn't do and comparing myself to others. Many times while practicing, I would catch myself thinking, *I can barely stay home for thirty minutes. How am I going to stay home for a few hours or a day?* When I told my therapist about my tendency to dwell on failure, he stressed the importance of learning to congratulate myself for every step forward. Patting myself on the back for every accomplishment, including the willingness to try, was an integral part of recovery because it increased self-confidence and self-esteem.

The tendency to compare myself to other people was just as self-destructive as berating myself. Sometimes while practicing, I thought about the people I knew who could stay home for days and weeks by themselves. I thought about friends who lived alone. While driving with Ellen, my thoughts strayed to truck drivers who drove across country by themselves. I looked enviously at women who were driving alone and thought, *Unlike me, I bet she can drive anywhere by herself. I bet most of these drivers take their freedom for granted.* I eventually realized that comparing myself to others in any aspect of life was harmful and irrelevant. I also realized that I did most of the comparing when I was frustrated with practicing and my slow rate of progress. I attributed my slow progress to the twenty-year gap between my first panic attack in 1967 to diagnosis and therapy in 1987. During that time without treatment, my avoidance behavior had become stubbornly entrenched.

By using distraction, positive self-talk and increasing the time I spent home alone in small, manageable increments, I progressed from five minutes to sixty minutes in about four months. It took focus and awareness to keep the feelings of panic at bay, but as I did so, I gained confidence in my ability to manage the hour at home successfully. I heard a tiny, new voice in my head that said, *See, you really can take care of yourself.*

Taking The Next Step-Driving Alone

After becoming comfortable with staying home alone for an hour while Ellen ran specific errands, I set out to accomplish my next goal. Rather than working solely on increasing my time home alone, I decided to practice driving alone from the flower shop to our house, a distance of about 2.5 miles. I approached driving with the same calculated steps that had already proven effective. My plan was to start with driving around the block then returning to the shop. After a few weeks, I increased my distance from the shop to home in one-to two-block increments. As with all practice, some days were easier than others. I took advantage of the good days by pushing myself further. On the bad days, I had to pull back. If I made significant progress on a good day, I knew I could repeat it.

The first time I made it all the way home, I couldn't get out of the car. I sat frozen in the driver's seat staring at the front door. For weeks I drove home, sat in the car for a few minutes then returned to work. When I couldn't get out of the car, my negative, confidence-eroding self-talk began: *What is wrong with me that I can't go into the house? Maybe I'm not ready to drive alone and be alone in the house. I'm so nervous from driving that I'm afraid I'll hyperventilate when I get into the house.* I had to counter these repetitive thoughts constantly. *I won't just hyperventilate instantly. I know how to control my breathing. There is nothing wrong with me just because I can't go into the house. I'm doing fine . Eventually, I will be able to go into the house. I have learned many new skills and I am determined to succeed. Maybe I can try to go into the house for a few minutes. I don't have to stay. There are always escapes and options. If things don't feel right, I can go back to the shop at any time. I am in control; my fears are not.* The power of choice, which allowed me to take charge of the way I practiced, made it easier for me to move forward.

After a few weeks of just sitting in the car, I ventured into the house. At first I could only stay for five minutes, but each week I increased the time until I reached an hour. As my confidence increased, I began to take different routes home. Expanding my route was the step that allowed me to begin driving around town by myself. Though I still couldn't stay home for more than an hour, I could see that it was a future possibility.

Finding Solace and Support in Group Therapy

The only people who knew about my panic disorder were Ellen, Dave and my therapist. I was still too ashamed to discuss the matter with anyone else, especially family members. I was not up to the misguided advice and demeaning criticism that my family might construe as help. I knew I was not the only person in the world with panic disorder, but this knowledge did little to relieve my feelings of loneliness and isolation. When I practiced, I felt encompassed by a surreal void that made me feel disconnected from the rest of the world. Given my belief that my feelings of isolation stemmed from a lack of contact with people who shared my plight, it was timely that my therapist started a panic disorder support group in 1988.

The group met in Sacramento. Ellen attended the meetings with me. Some members had been in therapy, but most had not. What a relief to hear other peoples' stories! I met men who couldn't work because they couldn't drive. There was a roofer who made appointments with people to provide bids or start projects. When the time came for him to go to his appointments, he would drive a few blocks, then return home. He was shaking and fighting back tears as he told the group that he could no longer support his family. By not showing up for bids and scheduled jobs, he had lost his credibility and his livelihood. He knew he needed help, but was too ashamed to talk about the problem. The men in the group had a difficult time asking for help. The women talked more freely about how panic attacks affected their lives. Some women could barely step out their front doors; others held down jobs but could not shop in stores or wait in lines. Several people were unable to drive on freeways.

One of the more unusual stories came from a middle-aged man who had been a packing shed manager for a large, national frozen food company. He was working in a windowless, claustrophobic shed when he had a panic attack, hyperventilated and passed out. Since he had panicked inside a stifling building, he avoided any enclosed place, including his house and car. As a result, he lived in his back yard, rode a motorcycle and became jobless. During the group meeting, he had to get up every few minutes to go outside because he couldn't stay in the room for long periods. He was desperate. He couldn't work and his wife was ready to divorce him. After his positive experience with group therapy, he entered individual therapy. Weeks later when I saw him in group, he was able to sit in the middle of the room without going outside, and what's more, he'd found a new job. The whole group cheered for him.

During my time with the group, I discovered that most people were embarrassed and ashamed about having panic disorder and were reluctant to confide in others. The majority had been either dismissed or misdiagnosed by doctors, adding to their fear, embarrassment and frustration. Everyone was relieved to know that there were other people with the same problem and that with the right help and practice, recovery was possible. Most importantly, in the group I was able to be honest, open and vulnerable, making it easier to talk about my fears and feelings. By sharing my feelings with others, I became part of the vast, human, connective experience that alleviates loneliness.

I was still seeing my therapist weekly and was now able to drive home and remain there comfortably for an hour, but no matter how hard I tried, I couldn't get past an hour. I was becoming tired and overwhelmed. I was working full-time in my business, attending chorus weekly and trying to change ingrained ways of thinking and behaving.

At my next session, I told the therapist that I was tired and discouraged and needed to either quit or take a break. He reminded me of how much I had accomplished. He also emphasized the need to be patient with myself because change doesn't happen all at once; it happens in plateaus. Regardless of his encouragement, I was tired of practicing and making weekly trips to Sacramento. Besides being tired and discouraged, I still had an oppressive fear of the big recovery picture. I continually thought about the hurdles that remained which undermined any feelings of accomplishment or progress. To ease the stress and frustration of it all, I quit therapy in the early part of 1989. Without the demands imposed by therapy, I felt temporarily relieved of my frightening commitment to change.

Return to Therapy

I took a year-long break from therapy. In that time, I neither regressed nor moved forward; I remained stuck. Eventually, I realized that to get past my stuck point of staying home alone for only an hour, I had to return to therapy. But I was reluctant to re-enter therapy because I was still afraid to do the hard work necessary to progress. Though my first therapist had helped me immensely, I was ready for a change. After much searching, I found a group of women therapists in Sacramento who specialized in the treatment of anxiety disorders. I contacted them and was referred to Nancy Lee. I began therapy again in May of 1990.

Miss Lee, who preferred to be called Nancy, emanated softness, kindness and compassion, making me feel welcome and comfortable. I determined that this would be my last attempt at therapy. If I didn't improve this time, I would have to look for another solution. I knew that medication was available for people with panic disorder and that psychiatrists could prescribe, but I had no desire to seek treatment with a psychiatrist. I had seen my mother under the care of three different psychiatrists and none of them had helped her. I found them aloof and uncommunicative, and believed that they only treated the sickest patients, the ones who ended up in psychiatric wards. Haunted by my mother's overdose, I had a deep fear of trying psychiatric medicine. So I naively hoped to overcome agoraphobia without medication.

Beginning Again

Since I already understood the basics of behavior modification, Nancy and I proceeded with goal-setting and practice techniques. My goal was to get past my previous limit of one hour at home and to extend the time to twelve hours. I committed to practicing three to four times a week, no matter how I felt. Even though I could already manage an hour alone, Nancy instructed me to start with staying home for just five minutes during the first week. Each week, I could only add five minutes to the practice time. I never altered the prescribed time. When I reached twenty minutes but knew I could stay longer, I didn't push past the allotted time. The same was true for bad days. If I had trouble staying home for twenty minutes, it was imperative that I remain home by using my coping skills. Again, the emphasis was on taking very small, manageable steps. By only adding five minutes a week to the time, I viewed each increase as tolerable. The recovery process is similar to escaping from quicksand; it is impossible to run out of the mire, you have to pull yourself out by inches.

As I succeeded weekly, my confidence increased. The challenge of increasing the practice time became an exciting contest, not an insurmountable chore. By the time I reached an hour, I trusted my ability to manage the anxiety. Instead of constantly worrying about how I could distract myself, I took pleasure in reading or sitting quietly in the yard. Since my time alone was now enjoyable, I began to look forward to it. I still had twinges of fear, anxiety and the occasional "what ifs," but they occurred less frequently and disappeared more quickly.

When I felt comfortable with an hour alone, I added ten minutes weekly to my practice time. I used positive, motivational self-talk often: *If I can stay home alone for an hour, I can do it for two or three. I have the skills and ability to manage by myself. Think about how good I'll feel when I accomplish my goal.* I progressed easily from one hour to two but had more difficulty getting to three. I was anxious to move quickly but had to be patient as I learned additional skills and more positive ways of thinking.

Learning to Value Myself

To continue with successful practicing, it was imperative that I learn to think differently about myself. Learning coping skills and practicing behavior changes were not enough. To become independent, I had to really believe I could take care of myself. I also had to learn how to recognize, respect and take care of my own physical and emotional needs.

From the time I was small, I believed that my needs were irrelevant. What was important and relevant was monitoring and caring for the emotional needs of my parents. There was neither protection nor escape from them. As I struggled to recover from agoraphobia, I began to realize that I couldn't waste my time or energy on my parents' ongoing problems. Every time I got caught up in one of their traumas, I became depressed and lost my practice momentum. I learned that my emotional survival depended on my ability to detach from their dysfunction. This was not easy to do. Nancy recommended that I set the terms of my relationship with my parents by determining both the amount of time spent with them and the acceptable topics of conversation. Setting limits and boundaries and sticking to them allowed me to be more in charge and less involved with my parents' unrelenting problems. Gradually, as I learned to pay attention to my needs and to trust my instincts, my depression decreased and I had more energy and focus for practice.

My therapist, believing in my ability to take care of myself and my desire to move forward, suggested that I set my own practice goals and determine the pace I would take to achieve them. She emphasized the importance of giving myself permission to trust and honor my feelings and to value myself by believing that I deserved to recover and to be happy.

Crossing A Barrier

By early 1991, I could stay home for three hours. By mid-1991, I had progressed to five. Getting from three hours to five was difficult, but I had learned that barriers and setbacks were to be expected and did not signal the end of progress. Though I was still plagued with doubt and discouragement, I viewed these disruptions as small annoyances. It was important to remain patient with myself and to be more optimistic about the outcome of my endeavors.

Once I reached five hours, the remaining time went faster. As 1991 ended, I had achieved my goal of staying home alone for twelve hours. Though I continued to use my relaxation tapes, positive self-talk and distraction techniques to manage my anxiety, a significant change occurred when I began to think differently about the fear. By taking small steps and staying in the feared situation until the fear passed, I learned that by facing the fear and flowing with it, I could overcome it. Every time I stayed with the fear, stared it down and got through it, I gained more control and strength. It now became clear that running from panic-producing situations or avoiding them had only reinforced the fear. Though my physical response to the fear remained real, practice taught me that I could change that response by changing my thoughts about the fear. With consistent practice, my dread of fear turned into anticipation of positive outcomes.

I had learned from both therapists that panic attacks have a short life span; they do not come and stay. If I felt myself spiraling into a panic attack and hyperventilation, I could use coping skills and wait until the sensation of panic wore itself out. Though panic and fear feel all-consuming and life-threatening, they are only temporary intrusions. Every time I flowed with the panic or faced down the fear, I became stronger.

The Positive Force of Anger

During one of my therapy sessions, I tearfully expressed my frustration with having to cope daily with agoraphobia. Though I had made considerable progress, there were many times when I felt overwhelmed and defeated by the struggle. When my therapist asked me, "Are you worth it?" I sat in stunned silence. I actually had to sit and think for some time before I answered with a feeble affirmative. I was distressed that I couldn't spontaneously respond with a hearty, "Sure, I'm worth it!" For days after this session, I was disturbed by my reluctance to champion myself. When I realized what little regard I had for myself, I became so angry that while sleeping, I often dreamed of hitting people. The intensity of my anger shocked me. I was mad that I had agoraphobia, mad at my parents and mad at myself.

It was as though a switch had been tripped and all my sadness and pain had been transformed into anger. While the sadness had evoked feelings of passivity and resignation, the anger gave me emotional energy. Anger restored the power and motivation to conquer my fears and improve my self-esteem. I focused on the things I could do, not on what I couldn't do. I never wanted to be a helpless victim again; I wanted to be in charge. Hopefully, the next time someone asks me, "Are you worth it?" I will respond without hesitation: "Sure, I'm worth it!" More importantly, I will believe it.

The Importance of Honesty

To be in charge of my life, it was imperative that I learn to clearly define my feelings. Since I couldn't readily access my feelings in most instances, I began asking myself, *What am I feeling now? Am I sad, happy, angry or afraid? How does a particular person or situation make me feel?* Many times I didn't know how I felt about encountering a person or situation until several hours or days afterward. Eventually, I was able to distinguish between positive and negative people and experiences. When I could better define my emotions, it became easier to draw boundaries with people, which helped me stop trying to please them or meet their unreasonable expectations. Once I realized that my feelings were allies and not something to ignore or be ashamed of, I could be more honest with myself and others.

Due to my high level of anxiety and a few bad medical experiences, for most of my life and to this day, I have feared going to dentists and doctors. I make appointments, then cancel them. When I do summon the nerve to keep an appointment, I am frozen with fear and sometimes cry during the appointment. I hate the helpless feeling of sitting captive in a dentist's chair or being shut inside a doctor's exam room waiting and waiting as the fear mounts. When I told my therapist about my fear of all things medical, she suggested I tell any health professional who would be caring for me that I had panic disorder. If I were honest with people, she explained, they could understand or accommodate my situation. When I got up the nerve to discuss my overwhelming fear of medical procedures with my dentist and doctor, I felt so awkward and vulnerable that I cried. But both of them responded with kindness and understanding. They assured me they would make any reasonable accommodations to alleviate my fear.

I told my dentist that one of my main fears was being trapped in the chair during a procedure. If I started to panic, I couldn't leave. After assuring me he could do a quick fix on my tooth so I could leave, he told me an interesting story about himself.

"I understand the feeling of being trapped in a seemingly inescapable situation. When I was a senior in dental school, I accepted an assignment of working on the teeth of prison inmates. To get to the prisoners, I had to pass through several locked metal gates and be escorted by guards down a maze of hallways. Every time I passed through a gate and heard it slam behind me, I felt a twinge of panic. By the time I reached the bowels of the prison, I had passed through five gates. With each of them locked behind me, I felt trapped and panicky. Once I got into the heart of the prison, there was no quick escape. As I did my dental work, I struggled to ignore the panicky feelings that kept intruding. When my work was finished and I was back outside, I felt an incredible relief. Had I known how torturous this assignment would be for me, I never would've accepted it. Anyway, my point in telling you this story is to let you know that I do understand what it feels like to be trapped and panicky and I'll do everything I can to make you comfortable."

What a relief to know that my dentist "got it." His willingness to share his story helped me feel less vulnerable and less reluctant to expose my feelings. When I first decided to be honest with my doctor and dentist, I feared that I would feel more vulnerable. Amazingly, the opposite occurred. Once I could identify and share my feelings, I lost my vulnerability. As I became a participant in my own health care, I took care of myself by setting up guidelines for my comfort. Now, before entering into a potentially anxiety-producing situation, I try to determine how I honestly feel about it and determine what I need to do to make myself comfortable. Once I was able to risk honesty, I saw how much I had underestimated other people. When I was reluctant to be honest, I deprived myself of their support.

I did encounter one doctor who demonstrated his indifference to my feelings by not responding to me. Since then, I just walk away from people who are indifferent or intolerant. When I am in control of my actions and choices, I have the power to walk away from any situation I deem intolerable. It takes practice to identify feelings and courage to share them, but honesty opens the door to more meaningful communication and relationships.

Phoenix

In the spring of 1992, my practicing routine came to a halt when Ellen decided to go to Phoenix, Arizona to visit her family. Her ninety-five-year-old mother, her sister and other relatives had moved from Ohio to Phoenix. Like the class reunion trip, I couldn't believe this was happening. I begged Ellen to postpone the trip until later, but due to her mother's age, she stood firm on her decision to go. Though I had made considerable progress with my recovery, I wasn't ready to stay home alone for two weeks.

After committing to go with Ellen, the next issue became the mode of transportation. Ellen wanted to fly, but after my Florida flight meltdown, I wasn't ready to get on a plane.

Driving was appealing because it was the only option that allowed for control and flexibility. Just discussing these plans struck terror in me, but I was determined to make the best of a situation I couldn't change.

My therapist helped me prepare for the trip. We worked together on visualizing the trip as I wanted it to be, not as I feared it might be. I made a list of things that would make traveling easier. I packed every form of portable distraction that room allowed. I took tapes, compact discs, crossword puzzles, novels and games. Ellen and I mapped out the entire route and figured the time and mileage between towns. Our plan was to drive six hours south to Ventura where we would spend the night. The following morning, we'd drive across the desert to Phoenix. When I saw the large expanse of isolated desert we had to cross, my mind imagined all sorts of horrors and the "what ifs" took hold. *What if the car stalls in the middle of the desert and we have to wait hours for help? What if I have a panic attack so severe that I can't continue the trip? What if Ellen gets ill on the way and needs an ambulance? I would be stranded in the middle of the desert.*

Though I made every effort to counter these thoughts with positive, realistic answers, I was unable to shake their menacing specter. After listening to my catastrophic ruminations, Ellen said, "Maybe the trip would be easier for you if a friend came with us. Having a third person along would give you additional security."

Fate took charge when I received a call from a friend who sat next to me in chorus and knew that I was fearful. As we talked and I imparted my fears and concerns about the trip, she suggested I might feel safer with a friend along. When I asked her if she could join us, she accepted. Now, I could quiet the "what ifs" by telling myself I had backup.

I maintained my fragile composure all the way to Ventura by employing the same strategies I used while practicing: I remained in the present, distracted myself and used my relaxation techniques. But the morning we were to leave Ventura for Phoenix, I was so apprehensive about crossing the desert, I cried during breakfast. I prayed for some unforeseen event to occur that might force us to return home.

When we arrived in Indio, one of the last outposts of California civilization, I had a full-blown panic attack. We had carefully calculated the time and mileage from Indio to Phoenix and concluded it would take about four hours to cross the desert. I had even called motel managers in Indio and Blythe to verify our calculations.

While we lunched at a restaurant in Indio, I asked the servers and the bartender the same question. "How many hours will it take us to get to Phoenix? We calculated four hours. Is that correct?"

The employees spoke in unison, "Oh no, honey! It's gonna take you at least six hours, maybe more, to get to Phoenix."

I was terrified to learn our calculations were at least two hours short. What seemed like a small error now became a major psychological defeat. I felt trapped and out of control. I started to cry. My heart raced and my breathing became difficult. With each moment, I became more desperate, feeling incapable of continuing the trip. I bolted from the table and went outside. As I tried to regain my composure, I started chastising myself for not using my coping skills to diffuse my fear before it escalated into panic.

As I sat crying in front of the restaurant, I felt like I wanted to die. I hoped Ellen would come out to tell me she was taking me home. I wanted someone to help me, but my out of control, irrational behavior created a communication barrier. While sitting alone in front of the restaurant in that godforsaken town, it dawned on me that Ellen could only offer consolation. She couldn't fix the problem. It was mine to fix. I was stuck with myself and it was up to me to adjust my thoughts and behavior.

With an empty stomach and a headache from crying, I climbed into the car and we started across the desert. The road was an unending straight line with nothing but sand and cacti on either side. The feeling of isolation I had only imagined became a reality. The road stretched for miles with no trace of civilization. The only signs of life were the other cars on the road. There were no gas stations, restaurants, bathrooms, or motels that could serve as a place of relief or comfort. The starkness and monotony of the road and scenery reminded me of an ugly setting from a science fiction movie. To distract me, Ellen and our friend Jane made conversation about anything and everything but the desert. I appreciated their normal conversation, but knew I had to keep working on myself.

To stop obsessing on the bleak terrain, I shut my eyes and listened to music. I knew that if I stayed focused on the road and mileage indicators, I would be stoking my fear and heading for disaster. I continually reminded myself to use the effective coping skills I had learned. I concentrated on breathing from my diaphragm and engaging in positive self-talk. When I employed these skills and stopped fighting my present circumstance, I relaxed long enough to realize I could manage my fear. Six hours after leaving Indio, I saw the skyline of Phoenix and felt like Dorothy gaping at the Emerald City.

Once we arrived and were settled in a hotel, I was relieved. Though I was more anxious than usual and longing to set foot back on home turf, the two weeks passed peacefully. Our travel companion entertained herself while Ellen and I visited her transplanted Ohio family. As the time drew near to return home, I started obsessing again on the drive across the desert. Ellen helped me when she said, "You've been across the desert once and survived it. But unlike the first time, you now know what to expect. This time, we'll be crossing the desert on the first leg of the trip, not the last, so you won't have days to dread it. Use your distractions and before you know it, we'll be in California."

On our departure morning, I planned six hours of distractions. Every time a negative thought intruded, I countered it with a positive one. When we stopped in Indio to have lunch at the restaurant where I had experienced the panic attack, I felt like a different person. The trip had made me realize it was my responsibility to make the best of my choice to accompany Ellen. To accomplish this, I was forced to employ every coping skill available to me. Though coping was a full-time job, in the stretch, I came through for both of us.

Resignation and Depression

After the Phoenix trip, I returned to my practice routine. Now that I'd given myself the freedom to drive from the flower shop to home at will, I was ready to tackle my next goal: driving around town by myself. Ellen, who had been a long-suffering support person throughout our relationship, was excited about the possibility of finally being able to run errands and to come and go by herself.

My therapist, Nancy, and I decided that I would start driving around town alone using the same methodical practice steps as before. To feel comfortable driving alone, I needed Ellen to remain in one spot while I practiced. She stayed either home or at the flower shop and I started driving the neighborhoods equidistant from those two spots. While practicing, I was tormented by the usual "what ifs" and self-doubts but I kept pushing forward.

I was making steady progress with my driving until February 1993, when at age 50, I needed a tonsillectomy. I blamed my father for this. During my adolescence, three

204

doctors had advised him to have my tonsils removed but he ignored them because of the cost. Once again, I had to deal with the consequence of his ignorant belief that doctors performed surgery solely for money.

As soon as I knew the surgery date, March 17, I began obsessing on the operation. My practice routine and forward motion came to another halt. The surgery went fine, but the day after surgery, Ellen's sister called to say that their mother was dying. Ellen found friends to stay with me and scheduled a flight to Arizona for the next morning. Though my throat was dreadfully sore and raspy, I managed to spend the day asking Ellen over and over, "How could you do this to me? I just had surgery and you're leaving me. You've never liked your mother. What if the plane crashes or you get stuck in Arizona? What would I do without you? I'm calling the surgeon to see if it's safe for me to go with you. I'd rather be miserable with you than miserable home without you."

"Look! You can call the surgeon but I'm sure he won't let you fly to Arizona. You're much better off at home. You need to rest. You'll be fine and I'll be back soon."

Though I knew Ellen was right, I called the surgeon anyway to get his opinion. After listening to my plight and my sobbing, he said emphatically, "You can't fly to Arizona. You just had throat surgery. You need to rest and take your pain medication. If you do too much, you run the risk of bleeding. If you started bleeding on the plane and were unable to get to a hospital, you could bleed to death. The risks are too high. You must stay home."

That night, I called my therapist in Sacramento, begging her to convince Ellen that she shouldn't leave. Instead, she tried to convince me that Ellen needed to see her mother. I was sobbing over the phone, pleading with my therapist to help me, telling her that I couldn't survive two days without Ellen. Over and over, she said, "You'll be fine. Two days will pass quickly and Ellen will be back. You have friends to help you. You may call me. Use your relaxation tapes and try not to catastrophize." At that moment, I was too terrified and inconsolable to absorb her advice.

That evening, while Ellen was packing, I carried on with the crying and pleading, incapable of rational thought or empathy for Ellen's difficult predicament.

When Ellen left the next morning, I was bereft. It was as if she'd died and I would never see her again. At that point, we had been together for seventeen years and had never spent a night apart. To maintain contact, she promised to call me at every opportunity. She called from the airports, her sister's house, restaurants and the hospital. She called every evening before going to bed. I spent the days looking forward to her calls and to my next dose of sleep-inducing pain medicine. With the amount of physical and emotional pain I was feeling, it was tempting to stay heavily sedated during Ellen's absence, but I felt the need to make some kind of contact with the friends who had graciously altered their lives to stay with me. To my surprise, when I interacted with them, the time went faster and I was able to disengage temporarily from my destructive thoughts.

When Ellen returned on March 21st, I was elated. But my euphoria was short-lived. On the day after Ellen's homecoming, her mother died. The funeral and burial were to take place in the family's home town of Columbus, Ohio. Ellen planned to leave for Ohio on the 23rd and return late on the 25th. I was so stunned I couldn't even sympathize with the loss of her mother. Putting distances in perspective, Arizona now seemed close and unthreatening compared to the flight-time and distance from California to Ohio. I honestly felt that I'd rather be dead than confront this situation. What was I going to do? Knowing that crying and pleading wouldn't work, I was stuck figuring out how to manage this new depressing and frightening reality.

The first thing I did was ask my best friend and college roommate, Susan, to come stay with me. Though she had just returned from a vacation in Hong Kong, she drove jet-lagged to our house from the Bay Area the night before Ellen's flight. The second thing I did was to give up the fight. Though the Ohio trip terrified me more than the Arizona trip, I forced myself to stop dwelling on disaster. My mind and body couldn't take it anymore. I was exhausted, sore, and tired from the tonsillectomy and the stress. I told myself, *Whatever happens, happens. I can't control Ellen nor any of the events surrounding her mother's death and funeral. To survive this situation, I have to believe that everything will be fine. My mind and body deserve a rest. Ellen deserves a rest from my neediness. If I love Ellen, I will support her as she has supported me. I know she'd rather be home with me but she needs to bury her mother. Listen to your tapes and think about the positive things you've learned in therapy. Practice resignation by giving it all a rest.* These were all the things I wanted to believe, even though they didn't flow naturally.

Ellen made it home as planned and we were both ecstatic. My time away from Ellen made me realize that I had taken her love and support for granted. I now had a new appreciation for her love, loyalty and willingness to give up many freedoms to help me reclaim mine. After my throat healed, I started to practice again. Compared with the tonsillectomy and Ellen's two trips, driving alone around town now seemed mundane.

By the end of 1993, I had made considerable progress with my practice routine. Ellen and I bought cell phones, and my phone became my lifeline. Just knowing that I could reach her any time decreased my anxiety and allowed me to advance more quickly. Besides working at our shop, I began exercising regularly and returned to my lifelong passion of painting. These activities helped me change my focus from the things I still couldn't do to the positive new things I was accomplishing.

Despite my progress, there was a darkness and heaviness that clung to me. I had felt this way on and off throughout my life but had tried to ignore it by presuming that it was an immutable part of me. But no matter how hard I tried to ignore this feeling, I couldn't shake it. I felt like Jacob Marley in *A Christmas Carol*, slogging up Scrooge's stairs encumbered by heavy chains. Now that this heaviness was getting worse, I felt forced to acknowledge its presence and determine its origin. When I discussed the matter with my therapist, she readily acknowledged that I was depressed. I had a difficult time accepting her diagnosis because my mother was the only depressed person I had seen up close and my behavior didn't resemble hers. My mother's depression had led her to alcohol, suicide threats, suicide attempts and two stints in the psych ward. But then I really didn't know how my mother had felt inside; I just saw the sad consequences of her feelings.

I asked my therapist why I was depressed and what I could do to fix it. Her response to the "why" included a combination of factors: genetic predisposition, family dynamics, distorted thinking and living with an anxiety disorder for twenty-five years. She suggested I should bring up the issue of antidepressant medicine with my family doctor or a psychiatrist and continue with talk therapy. With my distrust of psychiatrists and fear of psychogenic drugs still an issue, I wasn't ready to pursue that option, not even with my general practitioner. I continued my talk therapy with Nancy until early 1993 when I decided to quit. Though I missed my sessions with her, I needed another break from therapy and weekly trips to Sacramento. I spent the rest of that year continuing to practice, expanding my goals and trying to get up the nerve to contact my doctor about my depression.

In early 1994, I sat crying in my general practitioner's exam room telling her about the battle I had been waging daily to overcome agoraphobia and the heavy darkness that had settled in. She explained that many people with panic disorder also suffer from depression, and with the stroke of a pen, she gave me a prescription for the antidepressant drug Zoloft. Any fear that I previously had about taking psychogenic drugs was eclipsed by the more terrifying specter of depression.

After about six weeks on Zoloft, I felt wonderful. The darkness lifted, I was driving all over town by myself, I felt

209

light and full of energy, the gloom and pessimism vanished and I felt competent. I had either become a new person or the person I was intended to be without the depression. Then, after about seven months, my blood pressure became elevated, I had heart palpitations and a sustained rapid pulse-rate. Unfortunately, I had developed unmanageable side effects which forced me to discontinue the drug.

At the start of 1995, I had been Zoloft-free for several months and was sinking back into depression. At this point, I decided I needed a doctor who specialized in prescribing psychogenic drugs; I needed a psychiatrist.

Seeing A Psychiatrist

In early 1995, I made an appointment with a psychiatrist. As I wasn't comfortable asking around for references, I randomly picked a female psychiatrist out of the yellow pages. I based my choice on gender and well-defined ad content. Dr. Lumen's office was located within walking distance from my business, which meant no more weekly trips to Sacramento. Based on my experience with my mother's psychiatrists, I dreaded my initial meeting with her and insisted that Ellen accompany me for support. Luckily, after the meeting we both felt good about this doctor.

Since I'd long believed that psychiatrists were cold, remote and out of touch with reality, I was relieved to discover that Dr. Lumen (who at times I'll refer to as Dr. L.)was gentle, kind and welcoming. Regardless of her kind demeanor, after my first few sessions with her, I was somewhat uncomfortable and questioned my need to see a psychiatrist. I had been used to the more chatty, less formal structure of my previous therapy with non-MD therapists. Now, as I sat in my psychiatrist's office with books on Freud, Jung and other "Fathers of Psychiatry" staring at me, I felt that I had entered a more structured, cerebral dimension of therapy. At first, I was skeptical and intimidated by this new structure, but over time, I began to understand and appreciate the psychiatric model of therapy. I soon felt comfortable with Dr. Lumen and her collection of psychiatric reference material. In fact, I became intrigued by the science of psychiatry and its many facets and applications. I was also respectful of her intellect and many years of education.

The first few months were devoted to gathering background information and general assessment. I described everything I had learned from my previous therapists and the progress I had made through behavior modification. She reinforced the positive nature of the skills I had learned and praised me on my progress. I told her about my depression, my experience with Zoloft and my desire to move forward free of depression. The first antidepressant she prescribed produced the same negative side effects as the Zoloft, even in small amounts spread out over days. Over time, she tried several different antidepressants in varying doses and combinations, but every effort produced the same side effects: elevated blood pressure, heart palpitations and rapid pulse. My hope of being rescued from depression by a life-altering drug was dashed. As a result, I was relegated to talk therapy as an antidote.

During the first few years while I was trying different drugs, my therapy was focused on my early years of development and the part they might have played in creating my current state of anxiety, panic and depression. Since one of the Freudian interpretations of depression is "anger turned inward," one of my assignments was to write separate letters to my mother and father. This writing exercise was strictly for my benefit and would not be seen by either parent. At the time, I thought this was a useless, time-consuming endeavor. Regardless, I spent months writing the letters and reading my work weekly to Dr. Lumen. I was incredulous at the amount of anger that poured onto the pages. While writing the letter to my father, I developed a frozen shoulder, forcing me to spend weeks in physical therapy. This temporary shoulder impairment convinced me that childhood wounds and anger could cause physical as well as emotional symptoms. Though I wanted to quit working on the letters, I clearly saw that I had to purge the anger that had been festering inside for years. That anger, I was coming to understand, played a big role in my depression, anxiety and my habit of beating up on myself. This enlightening writing exercise solidified my respect for Dr. Lumen and convinced me that I had many lessons to learn and insights to gain from her wisdom.

I saw her weekly and continued to sort through the past while learning useful ways to identify and manage daily stressors. Unlike the focused, regimented practice therapy prescribed by my former therapists, my work with Dr. Lumen was focused less on a specific practice routine and more on my psyche, the deep inner self that gets buried over time by shame, fear, pain and denial. She guided me through labyrinths of painful emotions with the intention

214214214214

of leading me to growth through self-discovery and self-reliance.

One of the most powerful and painful exercises she occasionally assigned me was to get in touch with myself as a small child in an attempt to access how I felt when I was little and dependent. This is an emotionally painful exercise that takes much guidance, support, thought and practice. Every time I make contact with myself as a child, I cry for the sad and frightened little girl I see. I see myself as small but carrying the weight and worry of big problems and responsibilities. I sense my mother's fear of life, her insecurity, her neediness and her fear of my father. When these matters weighed on me in childhood, I felt the need to fix them. I didn't understand that fixing big problems was a job for responsible parents, not their children.

Every time I did this exercise, I had a better understanding of how I grew up to be a frightened and anxious adult. By becoming one with my little girl, I gained access to the developing core of my being. When I felt the sadness and pain of my childhood, I gained empathy for the girl I once was. When my responses to Dr. Lumen's questions sounded like words from a six-year old, I knew that my little girl was speaking. If I started to cry, Dr. L. drew me back in time to decipher the tears. Invariably, she asked me to put my arm around the little girl and comfort her. Sometimes I was perturbed with this request because I had no idea how to comfort anyone, let alone an invisible child. I had moments when I wanted to quit interacting with the little girl of the past and move on with current issues, but the girl wouldn't go away. When I tried to ignore her, she kept tugging on me, begging to be acknowledged, understood and comforted.

To maximize my forty-five minute sessions, I would make a list between sessions of topics I wanted to cover. If Dr. L. and I were working on a specific problem, I usually didn't get to the list. But when time allowed me to read my list, I rambled on breathlessly about all the topics I hoped to cover in a session. Sometimes my ramblings led to nothing, but usually they revealed some issue that needed exploration. This is when the psychiatric probing took place, a probing that took me further down the circuitous and sometimes painful road to self-discovery.

Before I figured out how psychiatry worked, I had expected the psychiatrist to supply me with the answers to every question raised by the probing. I was under the illusion that it was the psychiatrist's job to figure me out and to fix me, but sometimes when I asked her a question, she answered with a question. This left me stuck with both my question and hers bouncing around inside my head, trying to land on an answer. If the session ended before I could explore an answer with her, I left her office frustrated, knowing that I had a week to ponder the matter. At first, I found this technique of leaving me treading water dismissive and annoying, but as time passed, I realized that Dr. L. was teaching me to develop and trust my own problem-solving instincts. I was also developing insight, the ability to look inside myself and determine the true nature of a situation. I began to understand that the psychiatrist's methods were designed to teach me emotional resilience, self-awareness and self-reliance. Since it was impossible to develop these traits quickly, she became a patient, kind teacher, a listener and cheerleader—the kind of parent a child needs. Like a good parent, she knew when to take charge and guide me through a problem and when to let me find my own way.

Regularly seeing Dr. L. alleviated my depression. Just knowing that I could talk with her every week gave me the hope and energy necessary to keep me moving forward on a more positive track. Her steadfast presence in my life indicated her faith in my ability to become a functional person. It was my responsibility to internalize and practice her invaluable life lessons in order to become the person she believed in and the person I wanted to become.

PART FIVE
Letting Go

Alzheimer's: The Ultimate Challenge

In 1996, the year after my first appointment with the psychiatrist, it became apparent that my mother was losing her memory. She was seventy-eight and I was fifty-four. There had been random signs of forgetfulness several years before but nobody had put the pieces together. During that same year, my father, who was eighty, left home for good, moving in with one of his old girlfriends from high school who was also eighty. Both of my sons were still living with my parents, but planned to move out soon. Their departure would leave my mother alone. Robert, who was twenty-nine, had bought a house near my parents' and was working in financial services. Stephen, twenty-five, was planning to enroll in art school in San Francisco. I saw them often, usually when they appeared at the flower shop with my mother at lunchtime. Periodically, one or the other would call me aside to tell me, "There's something wrong with your mother. She's acting weird. Sometimes she forgets how to use the washer and dryer or puts things in strange places. She just acts confused. Whatever's wrong with her, it's getting worse. Maybe you should take her to a doctor." My father, who had power of attorney for her health care, created a document that allowed me to make health care decisions for my mother when he was unavailable.

Concerned about her symptoms, I took her to a primary care physician for an evaluation. In 1996, diagnosing Alzheimer's was largely a matter of ruling out other possible diseases. With the exception of a low mini-mental score, a test which measures cognitive impairment and is used to screen for dementia, and a brain scan that showed typical patterns of Alzheimer's damage, my mother was in perfect health. That, of course, is one of the cruel ironies of Alzheimer's disease.

The doctor's diagnosis was early stage Alzheimer's, but he wanted his diagnosis confirmed by the neurologist at the UCD Alzheimer's Clinic where the diagnostic accuracy rate is very high. Mom was evaluated by UCD in 1997 and diagnosed with mid-stage Alzheimer's. Up to that time, she was still driving, but during the family conference at UCD, we were informed that the clinic would notify the DMV and her license would be revoked. My father was also informed that my mother should not be left alone.

After the admonition from the Alzheimer's clinic, my father hired a woman to stay with my mother part-time during the day and early evening. Several days a week, the caregiver brought her to the flower shop to spend the day. My mother liked the employees and the constant activity in the shop. Though she had previously been able to answer the phone and wait on customers, she now busied herself with more simple tasks such as sweeping and folding towels. It was heartbreaking to watch my mother's brilliant mind waste away, but she was happy at the shop where she felt useful and could still entertain the employees with her humor. In the evenings, Ellen and I took her out to dinner or she dined with my sister or the caregiver. At night, when she took to sleeping in her clothes on the couch and leaving the doors unlocked, the caregiver began staying overnight.

My mother came to the shop from 1997 through 1999. By the end of 1999, she began wandering away from the store. When she disappeared, I never knew how long she had been gone or what direction she had headed. The surrounding shop owners knew her and called if she was in their store or had wandered by. Many times the delivery person had to drive around downtown looking for her or the employees took turns searching for her on foot. One time I was so desperate, I called the police to help in a search. My mother was strong and physically fit and could walk for miles without tiring; she had been playing tennis until she became sick. Unable to corral her any place in the shop, I was constantly on edge, leaping up from my desk every time I heard the store door buzzer. Though we always managed to locate her, I knew it was only a matter of time before something ugly happened. Now that it was no longer safe or responsible to bring her to the store, she spent her days home with the caregiver. After she stopped coming, I missed her terribly and knew that the good days with my mother were coming to an end.

One day in August of 1999, my mother walked away from her house between caregiver shifts. Though my father was not living at home, he still managed the upkeep of the home, participated in decisions concerning my mother and took care of her financially. In his attempt to conserve money, there was a gap in care between 7:00 and 8:00 A.M. When the caregiver arrived at 8:00, my mother was gone. On learning of my mother's disappearance, my father, my siblings and Ellen and I got into our cars and combed the area for her. When there was no sign of her, we called the police and highway patrol. Since nobody saw her leave, we couldn't provide a description of what she was wearing. When she was still missing in the mid-afternoon as the temperature rose to 101 degrees, the family sat huddled around the phone in my parents' kitchen waiting for some word from the authorities. By now, I had visions of her lying dead somewhere or of her crying, confused and alone, wondering where she was and how she got there. Then, there was the awful prospect of her still being lost at nightfall.

Around 4:30 that afternoon, the police called to tell us that a farmer had spotted a woman wandering around an orchard located about five miles from my parents' house. After much coaxing, the police got her into the car and brought her home. My mother, who had been gone for nine hours and had walked five miles from home wearing a coat, had no idea why everyone was concerned about her. Had she been less sturdy, she might have died from heat stroke, but she returned in good shape.

My mother's escape forced the family to consider what could be done to keep her safe. It would've been ideal for her to remain at home under the care of a loving husband, but that ideal didn't exist. After much consternation and contention, there was a half-hearted agreement among the family to place her in an Alzheimer's facility. The best facility available then was located in Citrus Heights, about forty-five minutes away. In April of 2000, my father took her there by himself. He made the arrangements for admission, packed her suitcase and told my mother that she had to temporarily relocate while major repairs were being done on the house. Despite the deterioration of my parents' relationship, my father was shaken by my mother's condition.

The family was instructed not to visit for two weeks after my mother's admission. This was an attempt to shift the patient's dependence from family to staff. During my first visit, I saw that my mother was lucid enough to know that she'd been confined against her wishes. "What's happening with the house? When can I go back home? I don't belong here. These are not my people and I'm not spending the rest of my life here. I want to be with my family."

No matter what reassuring words I could conjure up, she knew they were lies and that she was losing control over her mind and life.

Ellen and I visited her once or twice a week. At the end of each visit, my mother would beg us to take her home. Stuffed inside a dresser drawer, I found wads of lined paper on which she'd written both coherent and incoherent notes pleading to go back home. One comment she made remains burned into my memory. "I don't know why I'm here. I've never been a bad person. I don't deserve this." Nobody deserves Alzheimer's.

As my mother's disease progressed, I became overwhelmed by feelings of fear and sadness. Just driving into the parking lot of the care facility made me shaky and nauseous, reigniting the feelings of anxiety and panic I had fought so hard to extinguish. I dreaded entering the building and sifting through the blank, lost-looking patients to find my mother. Leaving the facility was just as painful as entering. My mother, who always tried to follow me out, had to be distracted while I punched the door code and guiltily escaped from her prison.

Along with my mother's diagnosis and confinement, sadness and dissension descended upon our family like a plague. Differences of opinion concerning my mother's care tore our family apart. Each of us was trying to do the best thing for mom, but we couldn't agree on a treatment plan. During a time when we needed each other the most, the family ended up dividing into camps, with one group barely speaking to the other.

Between my mother's deterioration and the ongoing, wrenching family conflict, I lost the energy and focus I needed to continue overcoming my panic disorder. Not only was I incapable of progressing, I began to regress. Things I could do previously without a second thought now caused me to panic. My moments of regression were not attached to any particular place or activity; they were spontaneous and unpredictable. When one of these panic attacks occurred, I temporarily avoided the place or situation that had made me uncomfortable. Though I realized that my mother's situation was causing me increased stress and anxiety in addition to lowering my emotional resilience, I became angry with myself for being unable to maintain my previous level of function.

Now in my sessions with Dr. Lumen, we focused on ways to deal with the family upheaval and my sadness and anger over my sporadic regression. She emphasized that the only behavior and feelings I could control were my own. Therefore, it was in my power to protect and care for myself. Though she acknowledged the devastating effects of Alzheimer's, she also stressed that I had no control over my mother's illness. She emphasized that the best way to help my mother was to take care of myself. If I lived in a state of sadness and defeat, it would interfere with my ability to visit and watch over my mother. Dr. L. reinforced the significance of the progress I had made and emphasized that temporary regression happens from time to time, especially during stressful periods.

With her insightful comments, Dr. L. kept me grounded and helped me see the potential for growth in difficult situations such as this one; but what was most helpful during this time was her calming presence that awaited me weekly.

During the summer of 2001, my mother collapsed from complications of a bladder infection. She was treated at a hospital in Davis and released to the Alzheimer's unit in an upscale retirement facility in Davis. Apart from my other feelings about my dad, I was grateful that he paid for my mother's care. With Mom now only three miles away, the stress of driving forty-five minutes on a crowded freeway was eliminated.

Adapting To Change

Ellen and I had been operating the flower shop together since 1977. Over the years, the shop had provided us with a good income and the opportunity to work together. By the year 2002, sales had started to decline while the cost of doing business kept rising. According to industry journals, many Main Street florists were losing sales to the ever-increasing competition from grocery stores and large retailers. Through buying power, our large competitors were able to sell flowers and plants for less than our wholesale cost for the same products. Realizing that this trend would affect our income, Ellen decided to return to nursing part-time.

Even though I could stay home alone comfortably for several hours, I was terrified by her decision to return to nursing. Being away from my support person was survivable when I had some control over the situation, such as being able to reach her by phone and knowing that she would be available to help me if necessary. But according to

Ellen, once she started working at the hospital, she would be much less accessible by phone and incapable of walking off her shift to help me. Her inaccessibility and my lack of control over the situation made me frightened and angry.

In February 2002, Ellen began working three evenings a week, 3:00 to 11:30, at our local hospital, which was seven minutes from home. Very rarely did she get off work on time. Emergencies, late admissions and loads of paper work often kept her there until 12:30 or 1:00 in the morning. Usually she would call during her dinner break to check on me and give me some idea of when she might be home. But her predictions were rarely accurate because of the constant change in hospital events. Sometimes, things in the hospital were so chaotic and demanding, she didn't even have time for dinner or a phone call. I was shocked to learn that on occasion, Ellen worked for ten hours without food or a break. On the nights when she was too busy to eat and came home too exhausted to eat, all I could think about was some poor plough horse that had been driven until it collapsed. If we had treated our employees that way, they would've quit or filed a complaint with the labor board.

Though I tried to be supportive of Ellen's decision to return to nursing, I couldn't overcome the anger and fear I felt about a decision which interfered with our somewhat predictable and comfortable routine. When we were working at the shop together, we had the freedom to come and go as we pleased. For example, many nights after work, we dined out, enjoying wine and conversation. When I wanted to visit my mother in the afternoon or evenings, Ellen always accompanied me to the Alzheimer's facility. Now, we had to work around a rigid hospital schedule.

At first, on the nights Ellen worked, I felt abandoned and anxious, and I obsessed on the possibility that I'd choke on my dinner with nobody around to help me. Many nights I simply wouldn't eat. Instead, I drank a food supplement. The old "what ifs" started again: *What if I pass out or have an accident and there's nobody here? What if Ellen gets attacked in the parking lot on her way to the car? What if I need Ellen and I can't reach her?* I tried my distraction and relaxation techniques but couldn't focus on anything except the clock and the countdown to the end of her shift. Though I was used to being asleep by 10:00 p.m., I now forced myself to stay awake until Ellen came home. I often fell asleep on top of the bed with my clothes on in case I had a panic attack or became so frightened that I had to drive to the hospital. My hatred of the hospital and Ellen's job was mushrooming. On the nights when she stayed past her shift, I was so angry I could feel my blood pressure rising by the minute.

After several months of blaming Ellen's demanding hospital job for my anxiety, depression and bad attitude, I realized that I had to take responsibility for my behavior and find my way back to rational thinking. Besides being angry with Ellen and the hospital, I was furious with myself for falling back into a state of helplessness I thought I had overcome.

I needed the help of Dr. Lumen to find my way back to rational thought. I was still seeing her weekly; I relied on her perspective and her ability to keep me on track. If I got off track, as I did with Ellen's job, her insight and guidance led me to a space where I could see the origin of my behavior and the solution to the problem. Many times, this meant a trip back into my past where I reexamined the self-sabotaging beliefs and consequent behaviors that continued to get in my way and derail my recovery.

There were three reasons I had such a negative reaction to Ellen's job: I had lost control of Ellen's constant accessibility; I believed that catastrophe would follow if I lost such control; and I believed that I was incapable of taking care of myself. Once again, Dr. L. emphasized that the only things I could control were myself and my reactions to life events. The idea that catastrophe would follow if I lost control was based on the distorted and erroneous assumption that I actually could control people and events. I had learned through behavior modification that the way to control catastrophic thoughts was to counter the negative thought with a rational one. To manage my time more constructively while Ellen was working, I returned to the lessons I had learned previously. Every time I started in with the "what ifs" such as, *I can't eat because I might choke.* I countered with, *I've eaten food my whole life and never choked. Chances of my choking are slim. I can always eat something soft. I will be fine.* In order to fall asleep while alone, I read in bed until I dozed off.

Returning to the basics of behavior modification over and over to get me through difficult situations was one way I could take care of myself. Though Dr. L. kept reinforcing the idea that I was perfectly capable of taking care of myself, it didn't always take. It was difficult to see myself as a capable, strong person when I had been plagued with anxiety, fear of panic attacks and in need of a support person since I was twenty-four. Also, when every new challenge threw me back into a regressive state, I questioned my ability to adapt and survive. Sometimes, survival didn't come naturally or easily like breathing; for me, it became a difficult, full-time job with no vacation in sight.

While trying to adapt to Ellen's return to nursing, I was also trying to adapt to my mother's deterioration. When Ellen first started working at the hospital in February, my mother was still physically strong and determined. Though she was living in the locked Alzheimer's unit, Ellen and I were permitted to take her out for walks around the large yard or have lunch or dinner in the facility's upscale dining room. Returning my mother to the locked unit was difficult. Every time I punched the door code to the unit, I felt like someone had punched me in the stomach. The stress of watching the essence of my mother disappear exacerbated the stress of adapting to Ellen's job. Most days, I could accept that at times my mother was walking around in dirty diapers or that she needed help eating, but sometimes, a single bad day at the Alzheimer's facility depressed me for days. Her smile when she saw me kept me returning to visit her almost daily.

While it was difficult to hang onto the practice techniques that kept me afloat, I forced myself to listen to my relaxation tapes consistently and to swim on a regular basis. These activities, combined with my weekly sessions with Dr. L., helped to make life more tolerable and my stress more manageable.

Grieving

In the late summer of 2002, my mother, who was now in a wheelchair, was transferred from the locked unit to the skilled nursing section of the facility. Though she had trouble speaking, she still recognized family and smiled when she saw one of us. She always had a big smile for my father who visited often. With her advanced memory loss, she had forgotten that he'd walked out on her.

My mother, now on hospice care, was visited regularly by the hospice nurses and chaplain. One day during the second week of February, 2003, the chaplain saw me sitting alone and crying in one of the parlors. She sat down next to me and asked, "Why are you crying? Is there anything I can help you with?"

I sobbed, "There's something that's been bothering me since the onset of my mother's illness. While my mother was still out and about, she used to come to my flower shop several days a week. She always carried a purse that contained a small, red coin purse. Inside the coin purse was a folded, beaten up article about Alzheimer's. Occasionally, I'd find her sitting on the office couch staring at the article."

The chaplain looked at me kindly as I continued. "Also, one time after the doctor had given her a mini-mental test, she started crying. After her appointment, I brought her home with me to distract her. But she wouldn't stop crying. She sat on the couch and sobbed. I put my arm around her and asked her why she was crying. Between her sobs, I caught the words, 'I don't understand anything. What's happening to me?' "

I stared at the floor. "Not knowing what to say and not wanting to say, 'Mom, you have Alzheimer's,' I said, 'You're all right, mom. You'll be fine. Don't worry. The doctor's just doing a routine exam.'"

The chaplain asked, "Did you ever sit down as a family and tell your mother she had Alzheimer's?"

"No, we didn't. We all agreed it would be better if she didn't know. Her biggest fear was that she'd end up like her mother, and we were afraid she might do something to herself if she knew. So none of us ever uttered the Alzheimer's word in front of her. We even told the doctors not to tell her."

The chaplain was quiet for a moment, then said, "Well, I think your mother knew she had Alzheimer's. That's why she cried after her mini-mental and read her newspaper article over and over. I think she wanted her family to tell her the truth. She wanted validation for what she already suspected. What do you think about what I'm telling you?"

"I think you're right. I've always had mixed feelings about our agreement not to tell her, but now I feel terrible that we weren't honest with her. She had a right to know, to be validated. I don't know who we were protecting, her or us. Maybe she would have eventually found peace in the truth, instead of fighting so hard against a disease she couldn't beat. Well, it's too late now. We missed our chance. She's too far gone to understand."

"How would you feel about telling your mother now? We don't really know how much she understands. Maybe by telling her, you and she might both find some peace. If you're not up to telling her, I'll do it. I see that your father and Ellen are here. Think about what you want to do. If you decide to do this, you need to explain the situation to your father. It would be nice if he were here when I talk to your mother. She always seems glad to see him."

The chaplain left the room to give me time to think. I was confused and terrified. I tried to think logically, but decided to go with my instinct. It seemed serendipitous that the chaplain had showed up while I was crying in the parlor and had encouraged me to talk. I decided that my mother still had a right to know what was happening to her, but knew I wasn't capable of telling her. I called my father into the parlor to tell him how I felt. He said, "I don't think your mother will understand what the woman says, but whatever you want to do is fine with me. I'll sit at the table with you, Ellen, your mother, and the chaplain when she tells her. Why don't you get the chaplain so we can get this over with?"

The five of us sat at a table and the chaplain began. "Hello, Mrs. Donato. How are you today? I am Barbara, a chaplain. I've visited with you before. Your family asked me to come here today to tell you something important. They want you to know that you have Alzheimer's disease. Your family loves you and will always be here. You don't have to fight anymore. You can let go. You can be at peace."

My mother didn't speak, but she was focused on the chaplain while she talked. When the chaplain finished, my mother looked intently at each of us. Then she smiled. In that smile, I caught a glimmer of gratitude, acceptance and peace. I felt more peaceful too.

The following week, on the morning of February 15, the day after a grueling Valentine's week at the flower shop, a force that I can only describe as telepathic, propelled me out of bed at 7:00 a.m. and led me to my mother. I arrived at breakfast time. My mother was sitting in her wheelchair at a table. The moment she saw me enter the room, she looked at me and collapsed, her head and shoulders falling to the table. It was almost as if she'd been waiting for someone from the family to come before she could begin the final process of letting go.

In the days that followed, family members had the chance to say good-bye. Before Mom slipped into unconsciousness, she also said her good-byes. She patted Ellen on the hand, she held my brother's hand during the night he stayed with her, and toward the end, she spontaneously opened her eyes and smiled at me and my sister. She died on the morning of February 17 with Ellen, my sister and me by her side. She was eighty-four and I was sixty-one.

Since my father was not there, the hospice nurse asked me to sign the papers to release my mother's body to the funeral home. When I stood there in a daze neither answering her question nor willing to leave the facility, she suggested that maybe I needed to spend some time with my mother's body; that perhaps I wasn't finished saying good-bye. When I told her I wasn't sure I could do that, she offered to sit with me for whatever length of time I needed. Trusting that a hospice nurse knew more about death and grieving than I did, Ellen and I followed her back into my mother's room.

As the owner of a flower shop, I had seen many corpses when I delivered casket pieces to funeral homes. But those deceased belonged to other families. Lying cosmetically treated in the casket, they had already made the transition from life to death. I had never watched someone die or seen the changes that took place immediately after death.

I was shocked at how fast my mother had physically transformed from life to death. Her skin had turned a strange yellow waxy color and her partially open blue eyes were cloudy. Her relaxed jaw had allowed her mouth to fall open. At first, I sat and stared in silence and disbelief. Then, I stood over my mother and sobbed. Finally, I got up the nerve to hold her lukewarm hand. While holding her hand, I kissed her on the forehead. Through my sobs, I told her repeatedly how much I loved her. I stayed with her for an hour. When I closed the door and looked at her for the last time, I knew she would be my protective angel and that I would see her again.

After I signed the papers to release her body, I thanked the nurse for gently encouraging me to sit with my mother's body. It became the first step in a long series of steps toward accepting and making peace with her death. It was the beginning of the arduous and painful task of grieving.

After my mother died, I felt lost. My entire body was weighed down by something indefinable. I lost my focus and I cried frequently. For months grief washed over me swiftly, unexpectedly and relentlessly. I cried in the most inconvenient places and situations. Anything could set me off: a song, a word, a smell. The list of triggers was endless. I felt anger, guilt and irrepressible sadness. I was burdened daily by an all-consuming anguish I couldn't shake. Though I didn't want to be around people; I was glad to be distracted by work, where sometimes I just sat in my office and cried. I worried that I was losing touch with reality, with only habit left to guide me through the motions of living. I feared that this new way of being might become a permanent state.

About six months after my mother's death, I was rescued from my private hell by an invitation from hospice to attend a six-week group session on grief. I gladly accepted, hoping I might find some explanation for my feelings. There were ten people and two grief therapists in the group. All the attendees had lost a close family member within the last six months. We filled out questionnaires about our feelings and we exchanged names and phone numbers. The therapists explained that the purpose of the sessions was to give the group an understanding of the nature of grief and its effect on the grieving.

In every session we received written material about the complicated process of grieving. We had homework to do weekly which each of us shared with the group. During the sessions, we were given time to talk about the deceased person and how the loss was affecting each of us. The therapists comforted us and validated our feelings.

I found the sessions invaluable. I learned that I was not going crazy and that my anguish, crying, anger and lack of focus, along with all the other new and disruptive feelings that surfaced, were a normal part of grieving. Though these feelings seemed unbearable and insurmountable at the time, I learned there were stages to grief and that the feelings of loss and pain would wane over time. I learned that grief was a process I couldn't fast-forward through; I had to live through it. Though everyone grieved differently and for different lengths of time, interacting with the group brought me out of my private despair and into a shared suffering. Sharing with others who respected and validated my feelings gave me hope, courage and the permission to grieve.

As time slowly passed, the heaviness of my grief lifted a little. I missed my mother terribly and knew that the missing would last until I died; but unlike the all-consuming and disruptive feeling of intense grief, missing was a feeling that did not interfere with my ability to function. I took solace in seeing her in dreams and feeling her presence everywhere. My mother's death gave me a different perspective on her life, and in the natural course of grieving, I thought about the many things I wished I'd told her while she was alive.

If given that imaginary second chance, I would have said, "Mom, I was never angry about your drinking. I understood your struggle with depression and the pain of your childhood. I understood how frightened you were and your need to cling to me. I wished you could've had a better life with someone who appreciated your brilliant mind, your eccentricities and your sense of humor. I'm so sorry you developed Alzheimer's. I know how much you feared ending up like your mother. I wish I could've taken care of you at home so you could have been with family. All you ever wanted was to be with your family. I know that you loved us deeply. I love you too and when you leave us behind, I'll miss you terribly. But I know you'll be someplace waiting to say, 'See, I told you I'd be waiting for you.'"

I spent the next two years, from 2003 to 2005, trying to return to the old normal: working at the store, driving around town alone and staying home alone. My efforts at all this were interrupted one morning in April of 2005 when my older son called to tell me that his father, my ex-husband, Dave, had died the previous night in his sleep. I was in my office when the call came. I started sobbing. Dave had been overweight with high-blood pressure for several years, but I thought he would be like his parents, who were chain-smokers and drinkers and had made it to their eighties. Dave was only sixty-four.

In the years immediately following our divorce in 1980, Dave and I had seen each other frequently. As time went on, our encounters became more sporadic. I attended a few parties where he was present and I occasionally met him at restaurants for dinner. Although he was married to his third wife, almost every time we were somewhere together, he drank too much and started talking about our marriage; he wished that we were still married; he was miserable without me; he still loved me; maybe we could get back together.

Every time I was with Dave, I felt the pull of our original attraction to each other. Being around him threw me into a state of confusion about my relationship with Ellen and the events of the past. On some level, I still loved him. After our divorce, I felt there were many things we had never discussed or resolved. I especially wished that we had worked on trying to save our marriage. I'd begged him to go to therapy with me. Once, in 1992, we actually had an appointment with a therapist but Dave backed out at the last minute. Now he was dead and I was left with many feelings to sort through.

After Dave's death, I became mired in guilt. I blamed myself for his death because I had left him and broken up our family. Maybe if we had stayed together, I told myself, he might not have wanted to annihilate himself by overeating and drinking. I was weighed down by regret, grief and the recurring question about my sexual orientation. Only after weeks of talking about these feelings with Dr. Lumen, could I begin to let go of them. She helped me realize that I was idealizing my marriage to Dave and reminded me that I had left him to be with Ellen for a reason. She also helped me understand that I was not responsible for Dave's death. Dave was a grown man who was responsible for himself and the way he chose to live. Even if Dave still loved me and longed for the past, it was up to him to find a way to move forward with his life.

Two months after Dave's death, I received a call from the coroner's office in San Francisco looking for Dave. His second wife, whom he had divorced to marry the third one, had been found dead in a cheap hotel room in San Francisco, and the coroner was looking for the next of kin. The conversation was unsettling. "Hello, I'm Dr. Smith from the San Francisco Coroner's Office. I'm calling you because I'm trying to locate the husband of Rachel Leigh and your last name came up as a match. Do you know how I can contact her husband?"

I said, "I'm sorry to tell you that he died in April and that he and Rachel were divorced."

"Well, do you know if she has any relatives I can contact to claim the body?"

"I know she has a son. The last I heard he was in southern California, but I don't even know his name."

"Well, we can only keep the body for a limited amount of time. If you find a contact, please give us a call. If nobody claims her body, she'll be disposed of as an indigent."

I told the coroner that I'd known Rachel and I wondered how she died. I also knew that she drank heavily.

He said, "When we found her she'd been dead for several days. There were a lot of empty vodka bottles in the room. That's all I can tell you. Again, if you find someone to claim the body, let us know as soon as possible."

He thanked me for cooperating and gave me his phone number. When I hung up, I felt sick. I felt bombarded by tragedy and death. I felt sadness for Rachel. I thought seriously about claiming her body and giving her a decent burial, but I didn't have the money or the emotional fortitude to pursue the matter.

After my mother's death, my father married Kate, the woman he'd been living with. When they married in 2003, both were eighty-seven. She moved into my parents' house after the wedding. They had two years of happiness before my father's death in September of 2005. He died a terribly painful death from a misdiagnosed kidney cancer that had metastasized to his spine. He had been having strange symptoms for five years, but his general practitioner hadn't seen a need to pursue them. He had been experiencing dizzy spells and on one occasion, was forced to pull onto the shoulder of the highway while driving home from Lake Tahoe.

My father and Kate were desperate for a diagnosis and treatment, but neither happened. A year before his death, Ellen and I took my father to several different doctors for a diagnosis. Kate always came along and ended up treating us to a nice dinner out after the appointments. Ellen and I liked her. She was a generous person with a positive attitude.

We visited my father and Kate regularly. When he was up to it, the four of us went out to dinner. During his painful illness, my father never complained. He was thankful for our visits and for the time we spent taking him to doctors.

When an internist finally did a scan, it showed cancer cells lighting up his body. My father's new doctor came over to the house to tell him about his diagnosis. Kate, Ellen, I and my siblings were there. The doctor said, "Mr. Donato,

I've come to discuss your diagnosis and what it means. You have cancer throughout your body. It started in one of your kidneys, probably a while ago. Kidney tumors are relatively slow-growing. If you had been diagnosed much earlier, the kidney could have been removed, preventing the cancer from spreading. There is nothing that can be done now. Your cancer is too advanced for treatment."

My father asked, "How long do I have to live?"

"You probably have a month to six weeks. I'm sorry to give you this diagnosis. I suggest you call hospice to help you with pain control."

When the doctor left, my father sat and stared, trying to absorb the magnitude of the doctor's pronouncement. He didn't cry, he just stared. Finally, he said, "Well, I guess that's it. The party's over."

Two days before his death was the first time I'd ever told my father that I loved him. He heard me and whispered back, "I love you too." That was the first and last time he ever uttered those words to me.

After Dad's death, I experienced a feeling that was different from grief. I suddenly realized I had no parents; I was now an orphan. I began dreaming about my parents several nights a week. In the dreams they were whole and happy. There were no bad times, just the fun times we had shared. When I awoke after those dreams, I couldn't believe that my parents were no longer here. When I worried about money or just felt lonely, I dreamed that if life became too hard or I ran out of money, I could always go back home. I saw myself being welcomed back into my parents' house and my old bedroom. Again, I awoke to rediscover that both the house and my parents were gone. After several of these dreams, I came to understand the meaning of the old saying, "You can never go home again."

From 2003 through 2005 I had been pummeled by death and grief. With the swiftness of Dave's death came the realization that life is fragile and fleeting. I learned from the good people at hospice that though the pain of grief ameliorates over time, the love for the deceased lives on. Though my pain has lessened with time, my mother, my father and Dave are always with me. Until we meet again, they stay alive in my memories and dreams.

In Retrospect

A few years after my parents died, I decided to sort through boxes of old pictures that needed to be put into new albums. I knew when I started the project that it would be painful, but I felt compelled to do it. By putting the pictures in chronological order, I could see the development of my parents' relationship as well as the fun times we all shared. The pictures taken during their courtship years of 1939 through 1940, show a handsome, happy couple. They married in 1941 and I was born in 1942. As the firstborn, I was the subject of my father's and aunt's compulsive picture-taking. There are several pictures with my parents dressed in their finest clothes holding me between them and smiling proudly. Like most newlyweds with a first child, my parents looked happy. In pictures of their early years together, they looked content. Looking at those pictures now, I have no doubt that my parents were in love.

In my late teens, after witnessing so much dysfunction, I wondered where the love between my parents had gone. How did their love and life unravel? I pondered over this question for years, both quietly in my mind and verbally in therapy.

There were many built-in impediments to the success of my parents' marriage. Just the difference in their backgrounds would've been enough to derail things. My father's parents, Angelo and Clora, were Italian. Angelo, who learned to make shoes as a boy in Naples, owned a popular shoe store in Woodland where he and Clora lived. Angelo, who could be jovial and charismatic, also had a violent temper. He had been orphaned as a boy in Italy after his mother died, and the family members who raised him had been abusive. As a teenager, he left Italy by himself to find a better life, but he brought his anger with him. If customers returned to complain about their handmade boots after they'd worn them through horse manure, he was known to throw the customers and the boots into the street with a warning not to return.

On Saturdays, when my father was out of school, he was expected to bring Angelo's lunch to him at the store. If my father arrived late, Angelo would beat him. My father always talked about the day Angelo sent him flying across the room when he was late with lunch. My father and his two older sisters were terrified of their father. Luckily, Clora who was much tougher than Angelo, didn't put up with his anger. When he started on a rampage, she'd banish him to the basement to cool off.

When my father graduated from high school, Angelo sent him to UC Berkeley. Two things were expected of my father after his graduation in 1938: He was expected to work in the shoe store with his father and to marry an

Italian girl. He accomplished the first, but not the second.

My father wasn't interested in marrying a bossy Italian woman who could cook and clean house. Instead, he fell in love with my mother, a blond beauty who was glad to become part of a large, extended family but showed no interest in becoming a domestic slave. Early in my parents' marriage, my mother's lack of interest in cooking and cleaning became a source of contention and criticism. Clora picked on my father for marrying someone who couldn't keep house, and she criticized my mother for being incompetent. After I was born, Clora insisted that my mother and I stay at her house so I could be cared for properly. This did nothing positive for my mother's self-esteem or self-confidence, which had already been damaged during her childhood.

When my mother fell into the world of Italians, she felt like a lonely alien. Angelo and Clora were hands-on people; they were doers and makers. They were smart, but they weren't bookish. My mother, on the other hand, came from a family of intellectuals. Both of her parents had college degrees, and her younger brother had gone through Stanford University and then Stanford Law School on a scholarship. My mother left college after two years to help support her mother, Selma, who we later called Besta.

The first time Angelo and Clora met Selma, they were awestruck. She was tall, with a stately bearing enhanced by her signature navy blue business suit. Unlike the Italians, she was soft-spoken. She was well-read and enjoyed lively discussions. She lived in an apartment in San Francisco and worked as a real estate agent. She didn't cook; she opened cans or ate at a diner. She never owned a home. After leaving her alcoholic husband, she had to manage by herself. There was nothing about her that resembled a 1940s homemaker. So when Selma and my mother became part of Angelo and Clora's world, it was a two-way culture shock.

As I continued sorting through the family pictures, I saw and remembered the good times. There was a photo of me that appeared in the local newspaper. I was six-years-old and dressed in full cowboy gear, perched in a saddle atop my dad's horse. I loved my dad's two horses; I used to beg him to lift me up so I could kiss their soft, smooth cheeks.

I found pictures of me on my first bike and many pictures from the late 1940s of me sitting on the shore at Lake Tahoe and swimming in the lake. In the early 50s, my parents took us to Death Valley, which we discovered was accurately named. The following summer, we went to Palm Springs where my father took a picture of us kids posing with Bing Crosby on a golf course. My dad believed in exposing us to different places and people. We were the first family in town to go to Disneyland. As kids, my parents took us to San Francisco regularly to visit our cousins and attend the 49er football games at the old Kezar Stadium. Every fall, we went to Cal games in Memorial Stadium on campus. Afterward, we'd eat at the famous Spenger's Restaurant in Berkeley. In the 60s, my parents took us to Hawaii, the 1960 winter Olympics and the Seattle Worlds' Fair. We were always on the go.

Then there were pictures of the parties. My parents had a heterogeneous mix of friends which made for lively parties. There were parties for everything: summer weekends,

Christmas, birthdays, graduations, wedding receptions, anniversaries and Fourth of July. We had a large backyard and some of the larger parties included 200 guests, a full bar and a band. I knew all my parents' friends and some of them were like family to me. They included some of the most eccentric people I've met to date. For instance, there was Marty, the law librarian, who once commented on a female guest's hairstyle. "She may have a beehive, but she's not my honey." Then there was Johnny, a Basque sheepherder, who frequently allowed his favorite horse to hang out in the living room when we visited.

My father learned how to throw a good party from his parents, who thought nothing of hosting twenty to thirty people for dinner. Clora, a gourmet cook, did most of the cooking with help from the other Italian women. Angelo barbecued on a fancy grill he'd invented which was the envy of his male friends. While the women worked in the kitchen, the men drank wine and smoked cigars on the patio. They all spoke Italian so I missed out on what they were saying. Because Angelo insisted that his children speak only English, the only time he and Clora spoke Italian was with their friends, when they were fighting or when they didn't want us kids to understand.

I found myself getting excited as I sifted through the box. I found programs from dinner shows we had attended at Harrah's in South Lake Tahoe and The Venetian Room at the Fairmont Hotel in San Francisco. In the 1950s and 1960s, famous entertainers performed in smaller, more intimate venues where the guests sat at reserved tables and ordered dinner before the show. My father always managed to get tickets close to the stage where we could almost touch the performers. Some of the artists we saw were Tony Bennett, Barbra Streisand, Liberace, The Mills Brothers and Louis Armstrong. My father, who was not shy, tried to track down the performer either during intermission or after the show to get an autograph. Amazingly, he nearly always succeeded. During Louis Armstrong's intermission, we followed my father into a hallway of the Fairmont where we found Mr. Armstrong. He graciously shook our hands and signed the program.

My mother had enriched our lives with books, humor and hugs, while my father had introduced us to people, parties, music, and the world that existed outside of Woodland. So how, with this seemingly ideal backdrop, did my parents' love and life unravel?

Though they came from extremely different backgrounds, they brought many of the same traits and problems to the marriage. They both had struggled with anxiety, fear, shame, lack of self-confidence and self-esteem, loneliness and depression. My father had expunged some of his anxiety by picking on my mother, vacuuming, cleaning house and washing windows. He was energetic by nature but driven into perpetual motion by anxiety. Alcohol and a good book had helped ease my mother's anxiety. My mother also had the additional burden of possibly inheriting the genetics of addiction along with the abnormal brain-wiring that some scientists believe causes panic disorder.

Though my father didn't appear depressed, the letters he left periodically on the piano were written by a depressed, lonely man. My parents both seemed lonely. Because they were fighting the same personal battles, they were incapable of comforting or empathizing with one another, which only increased their loneliness. And as their loneliness increased, they grew further apart.

Judging from the pictures of them in their early years of marriage, I believe my parents started out in love and happily optimistic about their future. Unfortunately, they were unable to recognize and overcome the problems that plagued their relationship.

During the middle stage of Alzheimer's, my mother struggled to apologize to me for drinking. At the time, I said, "It's all right, mom. I'm not angry about it. You were a good mom. You did the best you could, and I love you." I don't know if she understood me. She had already developed the blank stare of Alzheimer's.

Two months before my father died, he called me on the phone and said, "I'm sorry for the way it all went wrong between me and your mother. You kids didn't deserve that." It took a lot of courage for my father to call. I'd never heard him apologize for anything. I was so shocked, I didn't know what to say. So I said to him, "Thanks for calling, dad. I know we had hard times but we also had many good times. You and mom did the best you could. I appreciate all the good things you did for us."

In the end, before they let go, my parents were capable of recognizing the damage they'd done and asking for forgiveness.

Grave Matters

While reminiscing about the past, a disturbingly strange event came to mind. After Besta died in 1966, she was buried in Woodland's Catholic cemetery. My father had purchased four plots in the same row numbered 25 through 28, and they were intended for Angelo and Clora and my parents. But Besta died first and my mother wanted her buried in Woodland where she had enjoyed many good times and had spent the last years of her life. She wanted her to be close to the Italians and close to her own future resting place. My father had counted on Besta's sons to purchase a plot for her, but that discussion never happened. As a result, Besta, who had never owned a home, was now without a grave. To placate my mother, my father let Besta be buried in plot 28. My father decided he'd worry about the matter later, but as it turned out, the grave matter never became an issue for him.

In the late 1970s, after Angelo and Clora were already dead and buried in plots 25 and 26, Besta's son, a prominent lawyer in the San Francisco Bay Area, decided that Besta's remains should be buried in her family's plot in Steven's Point, Wisconsin. He reasoned that Besta would be happier lying next to her Scandinavian relatives. What he hadn't considered was that Besta had left the family farm years ago with no intention of returning. He had also failed to consider how exhuming and relocating Besta's remains would affect my mother.

One summer day in 1978, I received a frantic call from my mother. She was crying. When I answered the phone, I said, "What's the matter, Mom?"

"My brother Bob just called to tell me he's going to exhume Besta's grave and take her remains back to Wisconsin. I just can't take this. I've always been glad that mom was buried in Woodland. I'm the one who took care of her, not Bob, and I want her left alone. "

"Did you tell Bob how you feel?"

"It won't do any good. He's made up his mind to do this. He hardly paid attention to her when she was alive, and now he's decided to take her remains to Wisconsin? I don't understand his reasoning. He's just another man who thinks he can stomp all over other people. I guess that's what makes him a good lawyer. He's already talked to the cemetery and gotten the permit to open the grave. He plans to fly her remains to Wisconsin in his plane. I want you and Ellen to come over when all this is going on. I can't face this by myself. I've been through enough hell. I don't need this."

"That's fine, mom. We'll be there with you. I can't imagine how you must feel. This whole idea is really insane.

Just let me know what day this is happening and we'll pick you up. Is dad coming with you?"

"No. He doesn't want any part of this."

A few days after this conversation, my mother called to be picked up. When she got into the car, she was shaking. The cemetery was only two blocks from her house and we arrived before her brother. The grave was already open. There was no casket. All that was visible was a skeleton lying face up in the dirt. When my mother looked into the grave, she collapsed into tears. A mortician showed up with a wooden box the size of a suitcase. Some cemetery workers were standing around leaning on shovels by a backhoe tractor. When my uncle arrived, the mortician jumped down into the grave and started putting Besta's bones in the box. He carefully dusted off each bone before placing it in the box. When he got to the right femur, my mother pointed out the pin that was placed there when Besta had broken her hip.

My mother was sobbing and saying, "Poor mom. Her life was so hard. I'll be sad knowing that what's left of her isn't here anymore." Ellen and I were crying while trying to comfort my mother. My uncle, Bob, wasn't crying. He stood there tall and proud like he was still in the Marines. I just wanted the mortician to get the bones in the box so this horror show could end.

After the bone collection was completed, the mortician handed the box to my uncle. Bob took it to the car, got in, and drove away. All that was left was an empty hole in the ground and one in my mother's heart. We stood there as my mother stared into the hole while the cemetery workers waited to fill it in.

When my mother died in 2003, she was buried in plot 27, between Angelo and Besta's empty grave. At the time of my mother's burial, Besta's headstone was still in place on the empty grave. A few months later, the cemetery workers hauled it away and broke it into pieces. The only trace of Besta in the Woodland cemetery is now on the back of my mother's headstone where Besta's name is inscribed.

After my father died in 2005, he was buried next to my mother in plot 28, Besta's old resting place. It is ironic that during the time Besta lived with us, my father did his best to avoid her. Now, he was going to spend an eternity trying to rest in the same grave that Besta had occupied for twelve years.

"What are we going to do now?"

From 2006 through 2009, my energy was focused on trying to save the flower shop. Sales were declining, expenses were rising and the industry was changing fast. Hoping for a turnaround, Ellen and I borrowed a substantial amount on our home to keep the business afloat. By early 2009, as the general economy was spiraling downward, it became apparent that we were fighting an expensive, losing battle. We gave up our belief that with more time, the economy and our business would turn around. After spending forty years of my life in the flower business, Ellen and I closed the store on December 26, 2009.

In November of 2009, the month previous to the store closure, Ellen lost her job at the hospital. It appeared they were letting go of the older, highest paid nurses to make room for new graduates who would start at the bottom of the pay scale. Ellen had spent twenty-six years as a competent, well-respected nurse with a broad resume, and she loved her work. The day Ellen lost her job, she also lost big parts of herself: her identity, her self-esteem and her self-confidence. She struggled to hold it together, but she was devastated. With the job loss, I watched the essence of Ellen melt away.

Ellen was sad and I was mad. I had never liked what I saw of hospital policies and politics, but the way they'd treated Ellen was over the top. On the day she was fired, her unit manager called her at the flower shop to deliver the news. She lacked the fortitude and courtesy to talk to Ellen in person. To me, this was unacceptable behavior. I'd never worked for a large corporation so I had no idea how ruthless and uncaring they could be.

Ellen cried for three days, saying over and over, "I can't believe this has happened. I'm a good nurse. I've always had good evaluations and positive patient surveys. I can't believe the unit manager fired me over the phone. If I can stop crying long enough to get myself together, I'm going to make an appointment to talk with her in person. I've worked hard for that hospital and I deserve an explanation."

I encouraged Ellen to take action. "You're a good nurse and you don't deserve to be treated badly. I think you'd feel better if you could face her down in person. She's obviously a coward and probably hopes you'll just go away. Maybe you'll feel better if you take action. Besides, you're good on your feet. You perform well in confrontational situations." After a few days of crying and grieving, Ellen made an appointment with her manager.

After the meeting, Ellen gave me the rundown. "She told me I was fired 'for cause', which is a general term for incompetence. When I told her I had good evaluations and had never been written up for any reason, she explained nervously that there was at least one problem incident which she had discussed with me. I did remember the incident, but it wasn't remarkable." Ellen shook her head. "I told her I'd no reason to believe there was anything else negative in my file because nothing else had been brought to my attention. Then she commented that there were other issues in my file. When I asked to see the file, she refused to show it to me. Her final words were, 'We need to terminate this meeting. It's making me ill.' I walked away knowing that this meeting and the firing were a sham."

Ellen applied for unemployment but was refused because she'd been terminated. With encouragement from an employment attorney, Ellen filed an appeal. On the day of the hearing, Ellen and I went to the unemployment office together. I was allowed in the room during the hearing. Throughout the hearing, I watched the nurse-manager shuffle uneasily through her paperwork. She was unfocused and disorganized. Ellen stated her case clearly and convincingly. The unemployment judge granted Ellen her unemployment, overturning the original denial. With the judge ruling in her favor, Ellen had won a small, but financially important victory. As I watched the judge's face throughout the hearing, and saw the opposition fumbling for words and papers, I was convinced that Ellen had been a victim of some upper-management scheme to restructure the nursing staff.

With the store closing a month after Ellen's dismissal, we went through the painful process of emptying the store in a state of shock and disbelief. We had both been overcome by losses which challenged our fortitude. We were forced to reassess our lives. We asked the same question we had asked each other when we first decided to live together: "What are we going to do?"

With the loss of our two major sources of income, we could no longer afford our house payment. We had been living in the home we loved since 1981. Both the store and the house had served as havens where I felt safe from panic attacks. Now that the store was gone, I was left with only the house. I was so terrified by the thought of foreclosure that I continually catastrophized, picturing us living in our car or homeless shelters. After considering the ugly ramifications of losing our home, Ellen and I embarked on a ferocious campaign to save it.

For two months in early 2009, Ellen and I lived on the phone and computer looking for help. During this time, the country was in the middle of the financial crisis. The banks were consolidating and being encouraged to rectify the damage caused by bad lending practices. Our mortgage, which had been with Countrywide, now belonged to Bank of America. When we contacted B of A, we were two months behind on our house payment. The loan department suggested we apply for a loan modification based on financial hardship. Amid the mound of application paperwork, was a request for any hardship letters we wanted to provide.

On seeing the request for hardship letters, Ellen downloaded the entire ADA (Americans with Disabilities Act) to determine if there was anything relevant to panic disorder. Tucked away inside the large ADA document, was a section in Title II which addressed the rights of people with mental illness. With this hopeful information, Ellen and I put together a package of information for the bank. The package contained a letter from me explaining panic disorder and my subsequent need to remain in my home. My psychiatrist, Dr. Lumen, wrote a letter emphasizing that my mental health would be compromised if I lost my home. Also included in the package was the section from the ADA which discussed the rights of the mentally ill. Based on the information we provided, we applied for a loan modification. Within a week, the bank called to discuss the matter. Three weeks later, we negotiated a loan modification. Ellen and I were convinced that the ADA document had provided the impetus and leverage that motivated the bank to act in our favor.

Later, however, we discovered that neither the ADA document nor my panic disorder played a role in the bank's decision. We learned that there is no federal law requiring banks to consider the ADA guidelines for physical or mental illness when making loans. The bank decided in our favor because we were two months behind with payments and the government was scrutinizing the banks and implementing new lending practices.

Despair and Reprieve

After losing the store, I fell into an emotional abyss. I woke up every morning with no place to go and nothing to do. I bombarded myself with so many negative feelings I could barely get out of bed. I was sad, depressed, angry, defeated, regretful and fearful. Some mornings I would lie in bed thinking about ways to kill myself. Adding to my bleak emotional outlook was my dire financial situation. For the first time in my life, I had very little money. Even with the loan modification, Ellen and I were barely getting by on our combined Social Security checks. If one of us died, the survivor would be financially incapable of making the house payment and paying the bills. I obsessed on this terrifying scenario. I couldn't shake the fear of being homeless. I dwelled on the "what ifs" and "if onlys" and beat myself up for making bad decisions. *If only I had stayed with Dave, I'd be very wealthy. If only I had gone to a financial planner, I could have made better decisions. What if I do end up homeless? What would I do?* I even thought that losing the store was karmic retribution for leaving Dave.

Adding to my depression was Ellen's state of mind. She wanted to find a job, but after filling out many applications and getting only a few nonproductive interviews, she became depressed and discouraged. She was convinced that her age, sixty-eight, was a problem. I was surprised by the concept of age discrimination. One morning over breakfast, I said to Ellen, "I just can't accept that businesses won't hire older people. When we had the store, we hired lots of people in their sixties. They were the employees with the best people skills and work ethics. Besides, sixty-eight isn't old!"

"Well, I feel the discrimination when I walk in for an interview. As soon as the interviewer sees my gray hair, there is an immediate lack of interest in my resume. Now I know why older people dye their hair and get facelifts. I've talked to other nurses who lost their jobs when I did, and they're experiencing the same discrimination. They're dropping out of the work force and making do on their social security and retirement income. If I had stayed in nursing instead of working in the shop, I would have a retirement account. But I lost the potential for a good retirement income when I went with you to the shop."

While Ellen's mention of the shop as a negative force made me feel guilty for dragging her into the business, it also made me question my motive for jumping into the flower business after my divorce.

When Dave and I were discussing divorce, Ellen was working at the hospital, but I didn't have a job or a financial future. How was I going to manage? Dave was being supported by his parents and I knew with his history of ignoring financial obligations, I'd never see a dime of any spousal support. With my panic disorder, getting a job was inconceivable. The only option was to own and operate the flower shop in Davis. But I couldn't do this by myself. I couldn't even drive to Davis by myself. So I'd lured Ellen into the shop under false pretenses. I wasn't honest with Ellen or myself about how much I disliked the flower business. The arguments I used to convince her to join me in the business were true; if managed properly, the shop could provide a decent living, we could work together, and we could have more freedom. But I left out the part that my heart wasn't in the business: I was operating strictly out of fear.

When the business failed, I was forced to consider how my thinking and judgment was and still is distorted by panic disorder. Back in the early 1990s, before we borrowed on our house to downsize the business, the store was doing well. Our sales were the best they'd ever been and our debts were minimal. At this point, Ellen suggested, "I think we should consider selling the business. The rent will be going up and our sales are good. Now might be the best time to sell for a good price. We could pay off our house and I could go back to nursing."

Terrified by the prospect of Ellen returning to nursing, my emotional response was, "Why should we sell now? We're actually making decent money."

Ellen replied, "Well, I knew a wealthy businessman who bought and sold many businesses. He used to say, 'You always sell a business when it's doing well. You never know how long it'll stay that way and it's the time when you can

261

get the most money for it. But it's your business, you can do whatever you want."

From a financial perspective, I knew Ellen's suggestion to sell the business made sense. Unfortunately, I couldn't hear anything except the fearful self-talk in my head. *I'm comfortable at the flower shop with Ellen. If she goes back to the hospital, what am I going to do for a living? My safety and identity are connected to the shop. I'm afraid to go out on my own. I have to do whatever I can to make it possible to stay in the shop with Ellen. I'll think about selling the store when I'm not so fearful.*

As a result of this irrational thinking, I convinced myself and Ellen that if we downsized the store from 3000 sq.ft. to 1500, we could maintain our sales volume and decrease our expenses. We downsized in 2005, just before the economy went into a nose dive. Both Ellen and I were upset that we hadn't sold the business back in the 90s. We could have paid off our house and had a more secure financial future.

When I asked Ellen why she hadn't been more forceful in her attempt to convince me to sell, she said, "I felt like you needed to keep the business because of your panic disorder. I knew how terrified you were of losing someplace where you felt safe. I wished we could've had a more prolonged, deeper discussion about it, but I understood how frightened you were. I know you listen to people and are rational most of the time, but when your fears take over, you lose perspective. Sometimes, I become so enmeshed with you, I see things the way you do. And that makes me incapable of trusting myself and pursuing other solutions."

Ellen spent two years looking for a job that didn't exist.

To bring money in, I sold everything I owned that was salable: my jewelry, a large quantity of silver items that had been wedding gifts, and a beautiful grand piano my paternal aunt had given me. As much as Ellen and I tried to be optimistic, we lived in a state of fear and despair.

At the end of 2011, after Ellen had given up her search for a nursing position, my aunt died. Her estate was settled in early 2012, and I inherited enough money to get us through a year of house payments. The inheritance temporarily relieved the stress. Though Ellen and I knew the year would fly by rapidly, we were extremely grateful for the reprieve.

Pennies from Heaven

When my mother used to come to the flower shop during the time she was still functional, she and I would take walks around the downtown. Every time she found a penny on the sidewalk, she'd stop, pick it up, hand it to me and say, "Oh look, Di! Here's a bright, shiny penny. I'm giving it to you. It means good luck." Several times a week, we'd walk, she'd find pennies and give them to me. The penny routine became a ritual. I had a jar on my desk where I kept all the pennies she gave me. It was labeled "Pennies from Heaven."

During her time in the Alzheimer's facilities and after her death, I picked up every penny I found and cried. I always found a penny when I needed it the most and it brightened up my day. If I was depressed, the penny made me optimistic. If I was worried about some problem, the penny made me feel everything would turn out all right. I started to tape the pennies on paper and label the date I found each one along with whatever message I thought it was delivering. I even found a penny on 08/08/08.

What amazed me was that the pennies were always right in front of me, as if someone had planted them there on purpose. I'd find one right in front of a door I was entering, on the ground where I stepped out of a car or on the floor of a restaurant next to my seat. When I found one, I'd say to myself, *Hi mom! Thanks for the penny. I know you're watching over us and this is your way of being present.*

For three years after her death, I found pennies often. As the years passed, the penny sightings decreased. Now, thirteen years after her death, I often say to Ellen, "Where's my mom? I haven't found a penny in a while. She told me she'd never leave me." Soon after questioning her presence, I'd find a penny. I asked Ellen this question one night at a restaurant that had both indoor and outdoor seating. We were sitting inside by a window and when I looked out, there sat a penny on the patio next to my window seat. So whenever something encouraging comes along, like the following events, I give credit to my mother and the power of the penny.

When we received my aunt's inheritance, Ellen and I knew we were living on borrowed financial time. We searched our brains and closets for anything else we could sell in order to buy more time. Back in the 1970s, the flower shop had purchased an off-sale liquor license. The license allowed a customer to purchase a bottle of wine to include in an arrangement or a gift basket. At the time of our purchase, off-sale licenses were plentiful and inexpensive. As the big-box stores began sprouting up everywhere, each of them needed our type of license to sell wine and beer. With the demand for the license increasing and the availability decreasing, we were approached by a liquor license broker who had a buyer for the license. We sold it for enough money to make our house payments for another year.

With the financial reprieves maintaining us financially through 2013, Ellen decided to spend time looking for an internet job that would allow her to work from home. There was no shortage of "make money from home" schemes floating around the internet. Ellen looked into medical coding and veterinary assistant certificates she could earn from home. She called several insurance companies for information about getting hired as a phone advice nurse. Many of the legitimate programs involved extensive training, money and travel. At the recommendation of a friend, Ellen called a man who claimed to be just a step away from becoming a wealthy on-line entrepreneur. With this blowhard as her mentor, Ellen spent months on the computer looking at webinars where pitchmen gave testimonials about making thousands of dollars a month. After months of watching her waste time on these schemes, it dawned on me that Ellen could teach piano and music theory from home.

One evening, as she played some show tunes for relaxation, I asked her, "Why don't you teach piano? You're an excellent musician and teacher. You miss music and teaching piano would make you happy!"

She dropped her hands into her lap. "Ever since I lost my nursing job, I've no self-confidence. I'm afraid to put myself out there."

I said, "Teach kids and adults who are beginners. You don't have to teach university students who are majoring in music. Why don't you go to the music store and look at the books to get an idea of current beginner methods. Once you're familiar with the methods, get some signs for the car, put an ad in the paper and see what happens. You can put together a good resume with the amount of experience you have. If it works out, you'll get your self-confidence back doing something you enjoy."

I became a nag about this idea because I knew Ellen could do it. By late summer of 2013, she'd gotten up the nerve and interest to pursue teaching music. With many Davis people out of town for the summer, Ellen waited until school started to begin her ad campaign. The newspaper designed a simple, tasteful ad for her which appeared locally twice a week. She bought signs for the car and delivered flyers to local schools. By Christmas, she had several happy students and parents. And Ellen was happy!

Even with Ellen's starting piano income and our social security, we were going to have trouble making our house payment. We tried for another loan modification, but were denied. Once again, the bank paid no attention to the hardship letter written by Dr. Lumen explaining the need for me to stay in my house. The bank said over and over that they had no obligation to consider mental illness as a reason for giving us an affordable loan. Ellen and I called government agencies, local congressmen, mental health advocates and anyone who might be helpful. The answer was always the same: The bank has no obligation to consider mental illness when making a loan. We even went

267

to a well-respected real estate lawyer who wrote the bank a letter of opinion. He gave the bank a reasonable financial proposal that would work for us and the bank, but they weren't interested in making any accommodation. We were stuck with our unaffordable house payment.

Just when we started stressing again over the possibility of losing our house, my step-mother, Kate, died. My father had left his assets in a trust designed to take care of Kate through her lifetime. Although my father died in 2005 at age 89, Kate, who lived on martinis, made it until 2013. She was 97. In October of that year, I received my portion of the inheritance. I had hoped to invest the money, but it was needed for living expenses.

By early 2016, there were signs of hope peeking through the clouds. Ellen's roster of piano students was continuing to grow, along with our search for ways to increase our income. We were maintaining faith in ourselves and the power of the penny to get us to a more prosperous and peaceful time.

Mindfulness: Learning to Live in the Present

In 2016, I was seeing Dr. Lumen every other week. I was getting better about taking things in stride, but still had days where I felt depressed, sad and hopeless. I continued to worry about money and our house. I pictured us living in a car or a homeless shelter. I was disappointed that I hadn't made more progress eliminating many of my old fears and behaviors. I still couldn't fly or drive long distances with or without Ellen, and I couldn't stay home alone if Ellen left town. Neither of us had any freedom, which made us both feel badly for different reasons. Ellen resented her lack of freedom and I felt guilty and depressed for being responsible for holding her back. If I dwelled on this predicament too long, I thought about suicide as a way to free us both. When I got into this dark mood, Ellen reminded me that I'd come a long way from the days of sitting in the car in the hospital parking lot.

Though we couldn't travel long distances together or separately, I could stay home alone if Ellen wanted to do something in town. I encouraged her to go to a movie with a friend, join a social group, or engage in any local activity that would get her out of the house. I understood her need to make new friends and to create space between us.

In addition to my almost constant state of anxiety, one of my most annoying behaviors was my need to control everything. Almost every mundane movement had to be planned. If Ellen wanted to go to the Target store a few miles from our house, I'd say, "Can't you wait and go when we're going that direction? We'll be going that way tomorrow and you can go then." Most of the time, Ellen went along with my controlling logic, but occasionally she'd have a meltdown.

"Can't I ever just get in the car and go? What difference does it make whether I go to Target now or tomorrow? Do you have to control everything?"

I'd feel like a scoundrel and apologize. "I'm sorry. If you want to go now, go ahead. I just thought since we were going that way tomorrow, we could save gas." But she and I both knew that the issue had nothing to do with gas and everything to do with the control response I'd practiced for years to keep panic at bay.

I've worked hard to overcome my need to choreograph every errand. Unless I'm having a high anxiety day, I don't care where Ellen goes. On most days, she just picks up her keys and cell phone and says, "I'm going downtown to run a few errands. I'll be back in about an hour. I have my cell phone if you need to reach me." On the days when I can be indifferent to her leaving the house, I feel victorious.

During the forty years we've been together, Ellen has been a patient and loving mate. Though at times she has been justifiably frustrated and impatient, she has never belittled me nor minimized my illness. Whenever necessary, she has defended me. As part of the defense, she has tried to educate people who lack an informed understanding of mental illness.

Ellen's understanding and perspective on mental illness can be demonstrated by a discussion she had with a casual friend who said, "I don't understand how or why you put up with Diane's problem. If it were me, I would've dumped her a long time ago. I think you're co-dependent to her."

Ellen responded, "You've no idea what you're talking about. I love Diane. She's a good person and a good partner. I respect her. She has fought hard to overcome a difficult illness that took years to diagnose. I certainly don't consider myself co-dependent anymore than I would be co-dependent to a partner with cancer. When you live with someone you love who has an illness, you help them and support them, you don't dump them. That's the problem with so many people's perception of mental illness: If you're not crippled or suffering from cancer or another physical illness, then you're not sick or deserving of care and empathy. Most people don't understand mental illness. They think it's about being developmentally disabled or being a murderous psychopath. They think it's self-inflicted or a sign of weakness. Many mentally ill people have jobs, are functional and look like normal people. Mental illness isn't cured by slogans like 'Just get over it.' or 'Pull yourself up by your boot straps.' It's as serious and lethal as any physical disease."

I was shocked and delighted when Ellen told me what had happened. I was proud of her for having the loyalty and courage to stand up for me and the millions of people with mental illness who go unseen, unheard, misdiagnosed and misunderstood.

Driven by my need to understand how I ended up with panic disorder, I repeatedly asked Dr. Lumen, "Do you think panic disorder is the result of genetics or environment? Ellen had two panic attacks when she was younger, but she didn't develop panic disorder. I had one panic attack at age twenty-four and I've had panic disorder with agoraphobia for fifty years. In the books and articles I've read recently, much of the research on mental illness seems to point to brain wiring as the cause for many types of mental illness. Even though I spent my childhood with a fearful mother, I believe I was born with a brain wired for anxiety and fear and that's why it's been difficult to overcome my panic disorder. My brain needs to be re-wired. I also need to form new grooves in my brain to replace the fifty-year- old ones that are stuck replaying the tracks of anxiety and fear. Those deep grooves are the result of waiting too long for diagnosis and therapy."

Poor Dr. Lumen had to listen to my periodic rants about how backward the medical world was when it came to understanding the brain. Her usual response was, "I believe your panic disorder is the result of both environment and genetics. However, in the medical journals I read, there is growing belief that brain wiring plays a significant role in the development of mental illness. They just don't know enough yet. The brain is a very complex organ, and it may be years before they develop more effective ways to treat mental illness. Scientists are studying many new ways to treat depression and bipolar disorder. There are many potentially new treatments being studied, but until they are better understood and tested, we have to rely on traditional methods of treatment."

During my sessions with Dr. Lumen, I kept raising the old topics of depression, anxiety and my obsessive fear of being broke and homeless. Seeing that I continued to be caught in a destructive pattern of thinking, Dr. L. introduced me to mindfulness, a different approach to dealing with life and its inherent problems. Now she begins and ends each session by guiding me verbally through positive ways of being in the moment. During my sessions, she points out how I continue to sabotage myself by not staying in the present. She emphasizes that the "what if" scenarios I torture myself with have nothing to do with the present. The "what ifs" are catastrophic thoughts about the future, and the "if onlys" are thoughts about the past. Both modes of thinking do nothing but distract me from living life fully in the present. She addresses my obsessive worrying by reminding me that ruminating about problems does not solve them. She advises me to do whatever I can to solve a problem, then let it go. She encourages me to be grateful for what I have instead of dwelling on what I think is lacking.

In addition to practicing being in the moment, I'm learning the importance of being kind to myself by not letting thoughts and feelings define who I am. I can acknowledge and observe the feelings and either let them go or deal with them in a balanced, objective manner. Since feelings are transient, it is unproductive to dwell on them or give them power. By being in the moment, I can learn to differentiate between what is really happening in the present from any additional feelings I bring to the moment, such as projecting into the future or descending into the past. If I observe myself obsessing on a negative thought, I can break this cycle by returning to the present moment. While being quietly in the moment, it is easier to notice intrusive emotions and the bodily tensions they produce. When I feel tense, I scan my body to locate the tension. When I find any tension such as a clenched jaw or tight shoulders, I take a deep breath and let the tension drift away. If I can get out of the analyzing, judging and fixing mode and into the being present mode, I feel better.

Because I have spent years living with the "what ifs" of panic disorder, the practice of mindfulness has been a challenge. It takes awareness and persistent hard work to change entrenched ways of thinking and interpreting life events. Though staying in the moment takes effort, the practice of mindfulness makes sense to me. While practicing behavior modification, I learned that I couldn't be anxious and relaxed at the same time. The same theory applies to mindfulness: I can't be in the past or future if I am in the present.

Sometimes, when I'm practicing being in the moment, I'm drawn back into the past. Once again, I am the thirteen-year-old eighth grader sitting peacefully with Miss Simpson. We are working quietly together on a task and I am content. I feel her love and peace flowing through me. There is joy in the quiet moments we spend together. I know that she loves me and accepts me just the way I am. When it is time for me to leave for the day, I am sad. She knows I am going home to a sad place. Her parting words encourage me to be kind, helpful and accepting of my life at home. She gives me a gift by sharing her wisdom, her love and her ability to live peacefully in the moment. Unwittingly, at age thirteen, Miss Simpson introduces me to the peace and joy of being in the moment, the essence of mindfulness.

Many decades later, I find myself being content and peaceful sitting with Dr. Lumen while she guides me through my mindfulness practice. Like Miss Simpson, she teaches me that peace resides in accepting myself as I am and the moment as it is. She reminds me that life is neither perfect nor static and that recovery is an ongoing process. Consequently, it is important to learn, grow and be grateful for the simple things of the moment.

About the Author

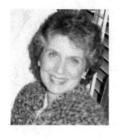 Diane Mengali lives in Davis, California. She graduated from the University of California, Davis, with a B.A. in English, and taught English at St. Francis high school in Sacramento for one year. From 1968 to the mid-1970s, she and her husband owned and operated Mengali's Florist in downtown Davis. After her divorce, Diane continued to operate the Davis store until 2009. Diane is an artist, and her work has appeared in many art shows in Northern California. Diane is a member of the local branch of NAMI, the National Alliance on Mental Illness.

To contact me, visit my website at: www.dianemengali.com

CPSIA information can be obtained
at www.ICGtesting.com
Printed in the USA
LVHW052257080622
720830LV00001B/128